central nerve plexus injury

central nerve plexus injury

thomas carlstedt
university college london, uk
& karolinska institutet, sweden

Imperial College Press

ICP

Published by

Imperial College Press
57 Shelton Street
Covent Garden
London WC2H 9HE

Distributed by

World Scientific Publishing Co. Pte. Ltd.
5 Toh Tuck Link, Singapore 596224
USA office: 27 Warren Street, Suite 401-402, Hackensack, NJ 07601
UK office: 57 Shelton Street, Covent Garden, London WC2H 9HE

British Library Cataloguing-in-Publication Data
A catalogue record for this book is available from the British Library.

CENTRAL NERVE PLEXUS INJURY

ISBN-13 978-1-86094-573-1
ISBN-10 1-86094-573-2

Typeset by Stallion Press
Email: enquiries@stallionpress.com

Printed in Singapore by World Scientific Printers (S) Pte Ltd

Contents

1

INTRODUCTION

Past and Present

This book is based on publications, as well as on materials from lectures and seminars for surgical registrars or trainees and from presentations for colleagues at conferences.

In contrast to a spinal cord or central nervous injury, a severed peripheral nerve can be repaired with functional return. Normality, however, cannot be expected subsequent to the repair of a nerve injury in the adult man. In most cases, brachial or lumbosacral plexus lesions are a combination of peripheral and central nervous system injuries. Therefore, they are the most devastating of the nerve lesions and also the most difficult to repair. Restoration of limb function and control of pain after such injuries are formidable and frustrating tasks. Prognosis for spontaneous recovery is often bleak, as there are several conditions under which recuperation is difficult.

Such injuries, located in the most proximal part of the peripheral nervous system (often within the spinal canal and close to the neuron cell body), can give rise to significant neuronal death. If regeneration takes place, the new neurites have to elongate for a long distance. They have to find their appropriate targets and form functional contacts without being sidetracked in the complex intrafascicular communications along the peripheral nerves. However, the most serious problem encountered in present cases of plexus injuries is when one or several spinal nerve roots have ruptured or have been avulsed (torn) from their attachment to the spinal cord (Bonney 1954; Narakas 1993). The root avulsion injury is a spinal cord (or central nervous) lesion, and therefore considered not amenable to treatment (Seddon 1975). It seems appropriate to consider those patients who have sustained plexus avulsion from the spinal cord as suffering from a longitudinal spinal cord injury.

Spinal nerve root or preganglionic injuries are a type of central nervous lesion, although the roots are, for the greater part, of peripheral nervous type. This kind of injury is considered impossible to repair with a functional outcome, as the regrowth of new nerve fibres has to occur to some extent within the spinal cord. Contemporary treatment is therefore palliative, using nerve transfers or neurotisations. Nearby nerves such as the accessory nerve, intercostal nerves, nerves from the cervical plexus, and even the phrenic or spinal nerves from the contralateral uninjured brachial plexus are used. In this approach, the interrupted connection between the spinal cord and the periphery is, to some extent, compensated for by alien nerves. But this is only palliative therapy; ultimately, the injured spinal cord segments will be permanently disconnected from the periphery, leading to secondary changes such as neuronal atrophy and death as well as giving rise to severe, excruciating pain.

The first description of root avulsion in brachial plexus injury was offered by Flaubert (1827) in a study of autopsy cases. The first exploration of a brachial plexus injury with root avulsions by means of laminectomy was performed by Frazier and Skillern (1911). Their case report still remains up to date, as it gives a clear description of the severe pain experienced by the patient after such a lesion and also advocates early intervention.

The first description of intraspinal root repair is of clinical cases of lower motoneuron lesions caused by tumours of the medullary conus in children with myelomeningocele (Carlsson and Sundin 1967). In some of the operated cases, there was functional restitution of bladder contraction by anastomosis of neighbouring sacral ventral roots. Thoughts on palliative nerve transfers from the upper part of the lumbar plexus were given later by Sundin (1972). Recently, descriptions of cauda equina repair after lumbosacral plexus lesion were published (Lang *et al.* 2004).

Direct reconstruction of the connections between the spinal cord and the nerves, after spinal nerve root injury, by implanting or re-attaching avulsed dorsal roots to the spinal cord, was first reported by Bonney and Jamieson (1979) in a case of brachial plexus lesion (Birch *et al.* 1998). The first human case of spinal cord reimplantation of avulsed ventral roots where functional recovery could be demonstrated was reported from the Karolinska Hospital in Stockholm (Carlstedt *et al.* 1995). Since then, intraspinal repair of brachial plexus injuries has been reported by other centres as well (Fournier *et al.* 2001; Bertelli and Ghizoni 2003). Recently, the procedure of intraspinal repair of lumbosacral plexus injuries (Lang *et al.* 2004) was successfully repeated in another centre (Tung *et al.* 2005).

Repair of the injured nerve plexus has always been subject to controversy. As early as the Roman times, the physician Galen was met with disbelief when he diagnosed a brachial plexus injury affecting hand function that he successfully treated in a nonsurgical manner (Robotti *et al.* 1995). Later, though initial great achievements had been made by brave surgeons at the beginning of the 20th century, surgical treatment came into disrepute and was abandoned for a long time. Early amputation of the arm used to be recommended. A more aggressive approach emerged with the development of microsurgery and the (overly optimistic) belief in its benefits. A new interest in these injuries arose, and has now led to the establishment of a paradigm for repair of the brachial plexus. The outcome of surgery is so encouraging today that it is no longer a question of what can be done, but of what should be done. Controversies, however, endure.

Thanks to the new molecular biology tools allowing us to explain the reactions of the nervous system to injury and subsequent regeneration, it has become obvious that an emergency operation is optimal for the repair of a nerve injury like a plexus lesion. However, this viewpoint is not adopted by all nerve surgeons. Another issue of debate is the approach to the most proximal of the plexus injuries, i.e. the root injuries or avulsions from the spinal cord. These preganglionic injuries have been considered impossible to repair (Seddon 1975), thus motivating the development of several palliative procedures (see Chapter 5). There is therefore a certain lack of interest in, and even some negligence towards, intraspinal injury to the extent that it is difficult to diagnose with certainty. The absence of surgical interest and exploration of such injuries has not fostered the knowledge in injury patterns, mechanisms, and surgical techniques.

After a rupture, the efferent or motor root would react as a peripheral nerve and, therefore, could give rise to functional recovery if repaired. Repair of severed ventral roots results in recovery of muscle function (Thulin and Carlsson 1969) and/or autonomic function (Kilvington 1907; Freeman 1949). In long series of animal experiments, the original idea (Carlstedt *et al.* 1986) of surgically treating the more central and frequently occurring avulsion of spinal nerve roots, i.e. the longitudinal spinal cord injury, was pursued for many years in the laboratory. The successful outcome of this intervention has been verified in several other laboratories (see review by Carlstedt 1997). This is the first successful instance of a spinal cord lesion where surgical treatment has led to useful functional return. Reimplantation of avulsed roots for the treatment of longitudinal spinal cord injury in plexus lesions has reached application in humans. The experimental background, the injury and its assessment, as well as descriptions of surgical techniques and outcome are here presented and discussed.

This book is also about ideas developed during early studies of the normal anatomy of the interface between the growth-promoting peripheral nervous system (PNS) and growth-inhibitory central nervous system (CNS) in the transitional region (TR) of the dorsal root, performed at the Karolinska Institute in Stockholm (laboratory of C-H Berthold) (Carlstedt 1977) and at McGill University in Montreal (laboratory of A. Aguayo), where the concept of spinal cord regeneration into peripheral nerve conduits was established (David and Aguayo 1981). The ideas were tested first experimentally, in collaboration with Staffan Cullheim, Mårten Risling, and Rolf Hallin; and were later translated to human clinical practice, in collaboration with Georg Noren at Neurosurgery, Karolinska Hospital, as the first step in treating a spinal cord injury, the longitudinal spinal cord lesion. Finally, some thoughts are given on future treatment of this particular lesion and related spinal cord injuries.

References

Bertelli JA, Ghizoni MF, Brachial plexus avulsion injury repairs with nerve transfers and nerve grafts directly implanted into the spinal cord yield partial recovery of shoulder and elbow movements, *Neurosurgery* **52**:1385–1390, 2003.

Birch R, Bonney G, Wynn Parry CB, *Surgical Disorders of the Peripheral Nerves*, Churchill Livingstone, London, 1998.

Bonney G, The value of axon responses in determining the site of lesion in traction injuries of the brachial plexus, *Brain* **77**:588–609, 1954.

Bonney G, Jamieson A, Reimplantation of C7 and C8. Communication au symposium sur le plexus brachial, *Int Microsurg* **1**:103–106, 1979.

Carlsson CA, Sundin T, Reconstruction of efferent pathways to the urinary bladder in a paraplegic child, *Rev Surg* **24**:73–77, 1967.

Carlstedt T, Observations on the morphology at the transition between the peripheral and the central nervous system in the cat, PhD thesis, Karolinska Institutet, Stockholm, Sweden, 1977.

Carlstedt T, Nerve fibre regeneration across the peripheral–central transitional zone, *J Anat* **190**:51–56, 1997.

Carlstedt T, Grane P, Hallin RG, Noren G, Return of function after spinal cord implantation of avulsed spinal nerve roots, *Lancet* **346**:1323–1325, 1995.

Carlstedt T, Linda H, Cullheim S, Risling M, Reinnervation of hind limb muscles after ventral root avulsion and implantation in the lumbar spinal cord of the adult rat, *Acta Physiol Scand* **128**:645–646, 1986.

David S, Aguayo A, Axonal elongation into peripheral nervous system "bridges" after central nervous system injury in adult rats, *Science* **214**:931–933, 1981.

Flaubert AC, Mémoire sur plusieurs cas de luxations dans lesquelles les efforts pour la réduction ont été suivis d'accidents graves, *Rep Gen Anat Physiol Pathol* **3**:55–79, 1827.

Fournier HD, Mercier P, Menei P, Lateral interscalenic multilevel oblique corpectomies to repair ventral root avulsions after brachial plexus injury in humans: anatomical study and first clinical experience, *J Neurosurg* **95**:202–207, 2001.

Frazier CH, Skillern PG, Supraclavicular subcutaneous lesion of the brachial plexus not associated with skeletal injuries, *JAMA* **57**:1957–1963, 1911.

Freeman LW, Functional regeneration of spinal nerve roots, *Quart Bull Indiana Univ Med Center* **11**:43–46, 1949.

Kilvington B, An investigation on the regeneration of nerves, with regard to surgical treatment of certain paralyses, *Br Med J* **1**:988–990, 1907.

Lang E, Borges J, Carlstedt T, Surgical treatment of lumbosacral plexus injuries, *J Neurosurg Spine* **1**:64–71, 2004.

Narakas AO, Lesions found when operating traction injuries of the brachial plexus, *Clin Neurol Neurosurg* **95**(Suppl):56–64, 1993.

Robotti E, Longhi P, Verna G, Bocchiotti G, Brachial plexus surgery. A historical perspective, *Hand Clin* **11**:517–532, 1995.

Seddon HJ, *Surgical Disorders of the Peripheral Nerves*, 2nd edn, Churchill Livingstone, Edinburgh, Scotland, 1975.

Sundin T, Reinnervation of the urinary bladder. An experimental study in cats, *Scand J Urol Nephrol* **17**(Suppl), 1972.

Thulin CA, Carlsson CA, Regeneration of transected ventral roots submitted to monomolecular filter tabulation (millipore). An experimental study in cats, *J Neurol Sci* **8**:485–505, 1969.

Tung TH, Martin DZ, Novak CB *et al.*, Nerve reconstruction in lumbosacral plexopathy, *J Neurosurg* **102**:86–91, 2005.

2

THE INTRASPINAL PLEXUS INJURY AND ITS NATURAL HISTORY

An intraspinal plexus lesion, a spinal nerve root rupture, or an avulsion from the spinal cord can be suspected in any patient with a history of high-energy trauma, such as a motor bike accident at high speed, in which the forequarter or hindquarter has been violently impacted and has become dislocated from the trunk.

The brachial plexus is little protected from traction forces because of the loose suspension of the shoulder girdle. In the most severe cases, particularly in forequarter dislocation, both the nerves and the major vessels are at risk. For instance, if the subclavian artery has been seriously injured — which happens in about 15% of these cases — and there is an abolition of the pulse in the arm, even if there is capillary refill, it is mandatory to perform vascular repair (cf. Birch *et al.* 1998).

Avulsion of at least one spinal nerve root of the brachial plexus (Fig. 1) occurs in about 70% of all brachial plexus lesions (Zorub *et al.* 1974; Narakas 1993). The lower roots of the plexus, i.e. C8 and T1, are more easily avulsed than the upper roots; C5–C7, because the latter are supported by ligaments at the exit of their foramina (see Chap. 3). However, traction forces strong enough to overcome those ligaments can cause complete C5-to-T1 intraspinal lesions. Tension in the various roots varies with the position of the arm at the time of trauma. Separation of the neck from the shoulder with the arm

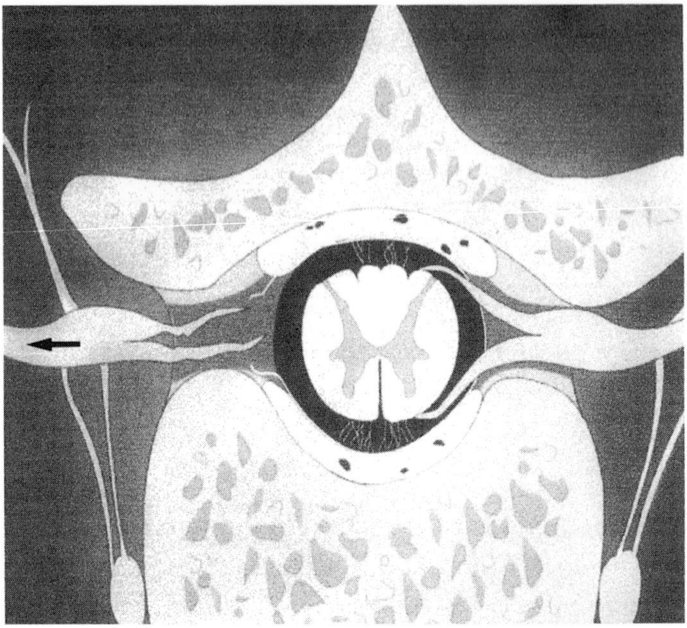

Fig. 1 Avulsion of spinal nerve roots. The connection between the central nervous system (CNS) in the spinal cord and the extensions in the nerve roots and peripheral nervous system (PNS) is interrupted. The arrow indicates the direction of traction according to the *peripheral mechanism* of avulsion injury. The roots and the dorsal root ganglion will be displaced out of the spinal canal (courtesy of Dr M. Risling).

hanging down will cause the largest traction force on the upper part of the plexus, i.e. the C5 and C6 spinal nerves and roots. With the arm in a horizontal plane, particularly in the case of an anterior-to-posterior directed impact, the middle part of the brachial plexus, especially C7, is at risk. If the arm is elevated, the lower roots C8 and T1 are subjected to the largest traction force.

Located within the bony pelvis, the lumbosacral plexus is more protected than the brachial plexus. However, in severe pelvic fractures, usually presenting as a dissociation of the sacroiliac joint together with fractures of the pubic bones, traction lesions can effect the lumbosacral plexus (Harris *et al.* 1973; Huittinen 1972; Huittinen and Slätis 1971) and its spinal nerve roots — the cauda equina (Eisenberg *et al.* 1972; Moschilla *et al.* 2001). Different mechanisms of injury have been described: flexion–abduction of the hip and posterior dislocation of the hip (Delmas *et al.* 1986), as well as hyperextension of the thigh with external rotation of the fractured and/or dislocated part of the pelvis (Finney and Wulfman 1960). In the case of fractures through the foramina of the sacrum, compression injury to the spinal nerves inside the sacral canal might occur (Huittinen 1972).

The spinal nerve root injury is a lesion where the nerves linking the spinal cord to the muscles under voluntary control, or to various sensory receptors in the skin or subcutaneous tissue, have been severed or avulsed (torn) from the spinal cord (Fig. 1). When both ventral and dorsal roots are engaged in the injury, the patient is subjected not only to paralysis, but also to sensory dysfunction (Bonney 1954; Narakas 1993) (Fig. 2). An excruciating, often unbearable, pain is almost inescapable after such injuries (Wynn Parry 1980). Therefore, the natural history in the adult includes the initial loss of motor and sensory functions in the pertinent extremity. The extremity becomes atrophic. The hand usually has a bluish-red tint due to paralysis of the autonomic nervous system. It is subjected to wounds and burns, as there is no protective sensation. Early, in many cases on the day of injury, the patient experiences severe, unbearable pain. The pain is typical, and forms part of the natural history after a root avulsion injury. It consists of two components: one is constant, e.g. a dull ache; and the other is intermittent, e.g. shooting jolts of a burning and compressing sensation (Wynn Parry 1980). The limb is often considered as a nuisance; in many cases, the patient requests to have the withered and painful arm amputated.

Other severe conditions could follow from spinal nerve root avulsions. Spinal cord tethering, or even herniation through the dural defect, can give rise to tardy Brown–Séquard syndrome and myelopathy with spastic paraplegia, which has been reported to occur late after the injury (Penfield 1949; Cilluffo and Miller 1980; Walter and Fairholm 2000; DaSilva *et al.* 2003). The onset of such symptoms ranged from 6 months to 37 years after root avulsion. Adhesions and arachnoid cysts, in some cases after a single root avulsion, caused compression of the spinal cord and interference with

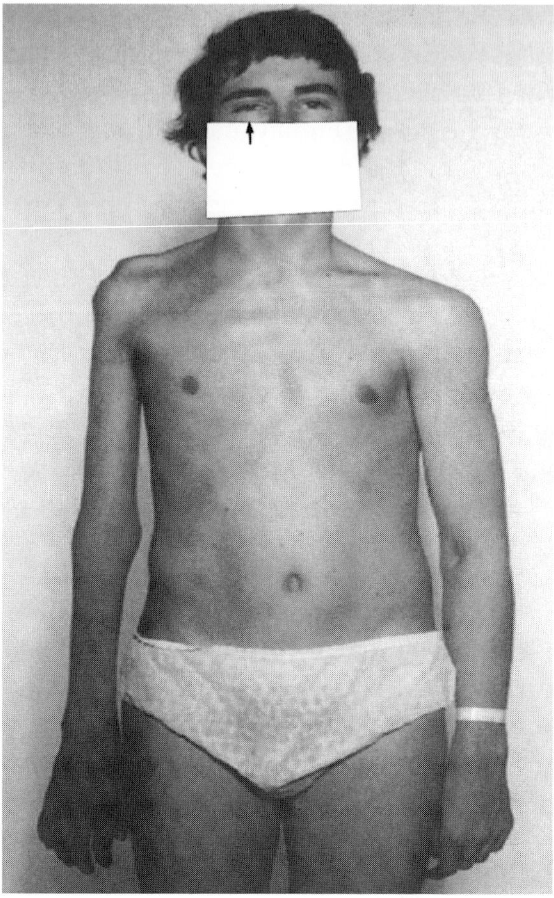

Fig. 2 Natural history after complete brachial plexus avulsion injury. There is an ipsilateral Horner's sign. There is severe wasting of the extremity and excruciating pain (courtesy of Mr R. Birch).

blood circulation, particularly chronic venous congestion, resulting in ischemic insults. Surgical decompression was followed by significant improvement of long tract symptoms, with arrest of progression of the motor dysfunction. Other rare phenomena that can occur late after the root avulsion injury include hemosiderosis, which can be progressive and fatal (Cohen-Gadol *et al.* 2004).

The natural history of the intraspinal lumbosacral plexus injury obviously depends on the type, extension, and severity of the nerve lesion. Persistent motor and sensory loss together with severe shooting pain indicate a severe injury with intraspinal root ruptures. Traction injuries can affect the lumbar part of the plexus with loss of function in the hip flexors and the knee extensors; they can also affect the sacral part of the plexus, with loss of abduction and stability in the hip, as well as paresis of the knee flexors and of the distal leg and foot muscles. If the lesion is most proximal in the lumbosacral plexus or affecting the cauda equina, serious disturbance to the visceral organs in the pelvis can occur as a result of a concomitant injury to the autonomic nervous system. Interference with bladder and bowel function leading to incontinence, as well as loss of sexual functions, can follow even from unilateral cauda equina lesions.

In autopsies, intraspinal or cauda equina lesions were observed to be quite frequently cases of ruptured roots. In contrast to traction injuries to the brachial plexus, avulsion of roots from the spinal cord did not occur (Fig. 3) (Huittinen 1972). If untreated, many patients are left with loss of function, sometimes accompanied by classical burning dysaesthesia and causalgia, for which management is difficult (Goodell 1966; Stoehr 1978).

In a peripheral nerve, the epineurium protects the nerve fibres from rupture. During a progressive stretch, the cross-section area within the nerve is reduced, causing an increase in intrafascicular pressure with ischemia due to capillary compression, and initial

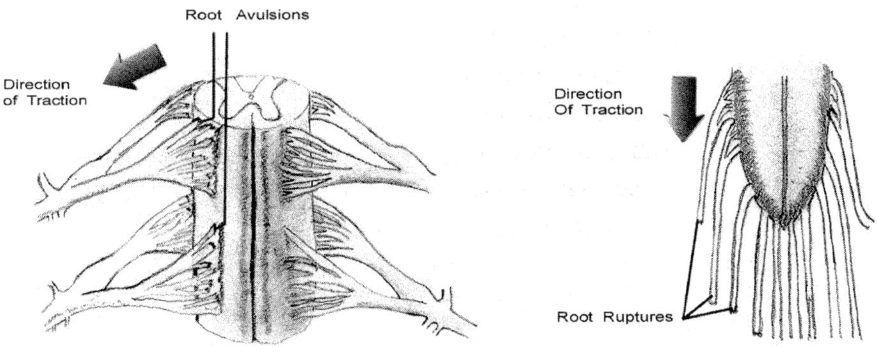

Fig. 3 Different injury mechanisms and intraspinal root lesions in the brachial and lumbosacral plexus (courtesy of Dr E. Lang).

nerve fibre damage. Further increase in traction will make the epineurium rupture, tearing the nerve fibres (Haftek 1970). Studies of stress–strain resistance showed that the maximum load before rupture of a root is about 10 times less than a nerve. Moreover, a ventral root is more fragile than a dorsal root (Sunderland and Bradley 1961), and the root–spinal cord junction is the weakest point of the root (Fig. 3) (Livesey and Fraher 1992). For these reasons, the roots are more likely to get avulsed from the spinal cord than to rupture when submitted to a severe traction force. Although a direct mechanical effect upon the spinal cord is unlikely, e.g. pieces of the spinal cord being pulled off together with the roots in severe traction injuries, such a lesion has been claimed to be responsible for about 10% of the cases of Brown–Séquard syndrome seen in these injuries. Anecdotes like these have been told in the surgical community without any substantial evidence from direct inspection of the spinal cord. In reality, long fibre tract symptoms are more probably an effect of ischemia from trauma-related compromised circulation (see Chap. 3). The tear happens at the PNS–CNS transitional region (Berthold and Carlstedt 1977), which makes this lesion a central nervous rather than a peripheral nervous injury. There is secondary degeneration along the proximal motoneuron axon and the distal sensory nerve fibres in the spinal cord following the trauma.

The root avulsion injury has also been called a preganglionic injury (Bonney 1954). Five different avulsion models have been described, referring to the transitional region as well as to the rupture of roots and if the dural sleeve is breached or not (Birch *et al.* 1998). With regard to the dorsal root, any lesion proximal to the dorsal root ganglion, be it in the peripheral or central nervous part of the root, is at present impossible to repair and must be considered in effect as a central nervous lesion (Carlstedt 1997). The situation is quite different in the ventral root, where any injury can be repaired with possibility of functional return. If there has been a rupture of the root, leaving a proximal stump of the ventral root still attached to the spinal cord, trophic support from the Schwann cells and other PNS cells ensures the survival of the motoneuron. This is a PNS lesion. A more serious, and unfortunately also more common, injury is the complete avulsion of the motor root through its central nervous part.

This will trigger a cascade of subcellular molecular events leading to rapid motoneuron cell death (Koliatsos *et al.* 1994). Repair is possible and can interfere with cell death, but it must be done urgently.

Within each injured plexus, there are considerable variations in the type of root lesion (Carlstedt *et al.* 2000; Carvalho *et al.* 1997; Privat *et al.* 1982). There is a combination of total and partial ruptures and avulsions, leaving either the dorsal or the ventral root intact (see Chap. 4, Fig. 9). The most frequent pattern is complete avulsion of dorsal and ventral roots, mostly of the lower roots of the brachial plexus, C8 and T1. The combination of intact dorsal and avulsed ventral roots is more common than spared ventral and torn dorsal root. Most of the partial root avulsions concern the upper nerves of the plexus, C5 and C6 (Carlstedt and Noren 1995; Carlstedt *et al.* 1995; Birch *et al.* 1998).

Although the exact process leading to root avulsion is not completely understood, two mechanisms have been described. The *peripheral mechanism* (Fig. 1) is a lateral or peripheral traction force onto the root and spinal nerve that, when forceful enough, pulls the roots off the spinal cord while displacing the ganglion out of the intervertebral foramen [Figs. 4(b) and 5(a)] (Mansat 1977; Mansat *et al.* 1979). This is prevalent in adult trauma cases. After such a traction, the roots and the ganglion can be found in between the scaleni muscles or, even further distally, underneath the clavicle. In the *central mechanism*, the roots have been detached from the spinal cord, but the ganglion and the roots have not been displaced out of the spinal canal or the foramen [Figs. 4(a) and 5(b)]. This paradoxical situation is thought to depend on an axial rather than a lateral force, occurring during a shift in the spinal cord from an excessive lateral flexion of the spinal cord (Sunderland 1974). By the excessive lateral flexion of the neck, the spinal cord pulls in cranial direction away from the roots that are anchored at the intervertebral foramina. This type of root avulsion is likely to occur when there has been an impact to the cervical spine, sometimes with vertebral fractures, rather than a trauma to the shoulder.

A mixture of a peripheral and central mechanism of root avulsion can sometimes be seen when exposing the spinal canal [Fig. 5(b)]. This type of injury is probably most common in obstetric brachial

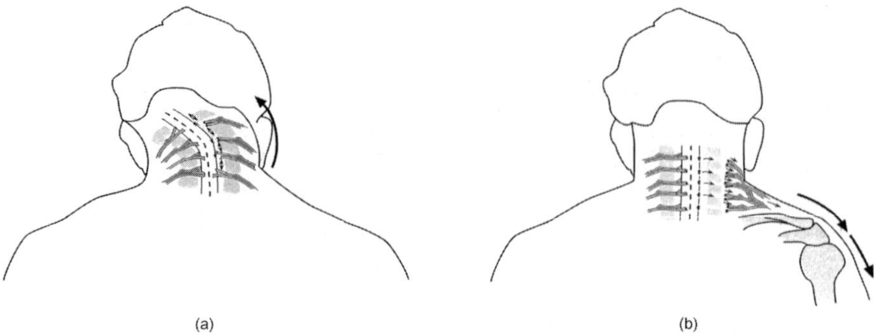

Fig. 4 Root avulsions. The (a) central and (b) peripheral mechanisms of root avulsion. (a) In lateral flexion of the spine and spinal cord (large arrow), there is a longitudinal shearing force that separates the roots from their attachments with the spinal cord without displacement out of the spinal canal. The spinal cord is pulled in a cranial direction in relation to the spine, whereas the roots are held by the spine and their attachments to the intervertebral foramina (small arrows). (b) The loose suspension of the shoulder girdle makes the brachial plexus particularly susceptible to traction injury when there is a trauma that separates the shoulder from the neck (large arrows). Root avulsion with lateral displacement of the spinal nerve roots out of the spinal canal (small arrows) occurs if the force is of sufficient magnitude.

plexus injuries, when shoulder dystocia necessitates excessive lateral flexion of the neck. From an extraspinal exploration of the posterior triangle of the neck, one can get the false impression of an uninjured plexus, with spinal nerves *in situ* up to the foramina. It is difficult to give a certain diagnosis for this kind of severe intraspinal lesion. Preoperative scanning is often unable to show signs of root avulsion, such as pseudomeningoceles, as the dura is not torn in the injury. Even if preoperative electrophysiology (SSEP) is used, there might still be parts of the dorsal root more resistant to traction injury than the ventral root, which remain in continuity with the spinal cord, thus giving a "false" response. Several diagnostic mistakes and wrong treatments in adults, but mainly in children with obstetrical brachial plexus lesion, occur in this situation (see Chap. 4).

Ruptures of the spinal nerves within the intervertebral canal are a less described type of injury (Kline *et al.* 1992; Carlstedt and Noren

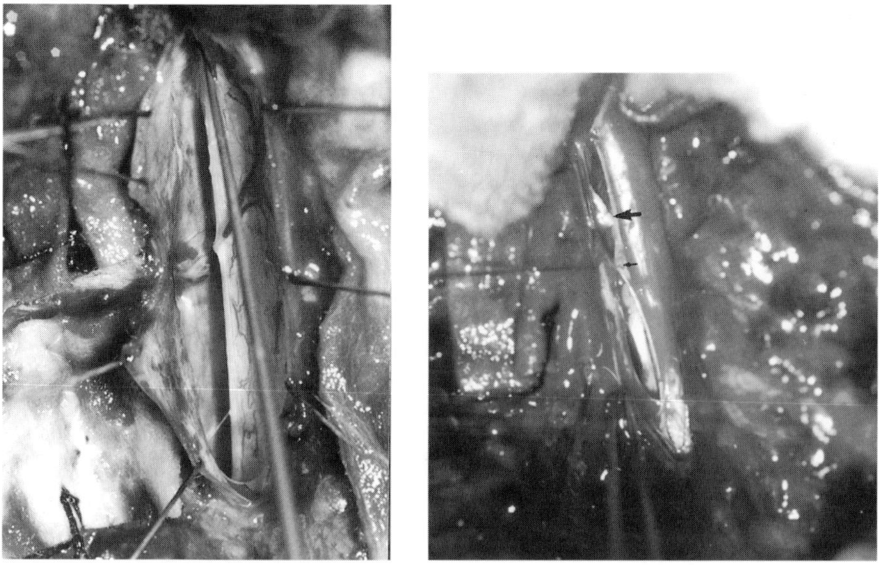

(a) (b)

Fig. 5 Intraspinal exposure of root avulsions. (a) Complete avulsions with empty internal foramen. (b) Intact denticulate attachment (small arrow). A root which has been avulsed but still rests within the subdural space can be seen (arrow) (from Carlstedt *et al.* 2000).

1995). These sometimes appear as most proximal spinal nerve ruptures distal to the ganglion (Kline *et al.* 1992). A "classical" nerve graft repair is possible in such cases. However, if the rupture is situated in the proximal part of the intervertebral canal and is preganglionic, then the injury is still possible to repair but only for motor recovery (Carlstedt and Noren 1995). This type of injury can be the result of a forceful traction in the upper part of the plexus, but they more often occur as a consequence of direct impact to the base of the neck, in cases of C8–T1 involvement (Carlstedt and Noren 1995).

Finally, the bilateral brachial plexus lesion is more common after birth trauma than in the adult. This type of injury can happen in the adult when the patient is injured by repetitive impacts or in a blast:

Case. A 19-year-old male working in a shipyard was sandblasting a boat, when the pressure container holding the sand exploded as he was standing on its top. He was propelled about 10 m up in the air from the blast. He had immediate loss of bilateral upper extremity motor and sensory function. An MRI and CT myelogram showed avulsion injuries with roots present on the right side only for C5, and on the left side at C5 and also a ventral root at C6. There was clinically no function in the right arm; but some spared muscle function on the left side for the supraspinatus, the deltoid, and the triceps. There were no neurological deficits in his lower extremities. He had an extraspinal and intraspinal exploration of his brachial plexus injuries. On the right side, there was a ruptured C5 with a stump that also received a contribution from C4, i.e. a prefixed plexus. A small stump was also found for C6. Intraspinal exploration revealed an intact ventral root at C5 and some remnants of the C6 ventral root extending out through the foramen. The roots C7–T1 were all avulsed from the spinal cord. On the left side, there were only ruptured stumps of C5 and C6. C7 to T1 appeared avulsed from the spinal cord.

In a comprehensive review, Huittinen (1972) and Huittinen and Slätis (1971) reported that in approximately half of the patients presenting persistent neurological symptoms after pelvic fractures with sacroiliac joint dislocations, there were ruptures of the lumbosacral roots L3–S3, in some cases bilaterally. No avulsion from the spinal cord was observed. This reflects the different mechanisms involved. Injuries to cervical roots to the brachial plexus are due to a nearly horizontal traction, causing avulsions from the spinal cord. The traction applied to the lumbosacral nerve roots (e.g. in pelvic fractures) is almost parallel to the long axis of the spinal cord. Therefore, the roots rupture along their course intradurally, but proximal to the spinal ganglion and distal to their origin from the lumbar enlargement of the spinal cord (Fig. 3). Thus, nerve root avulsion of roots in the cauda equina is rare (Barnett and Connolly 1975).

Conclusion

The most severe plexus injuries are associated with intraspinal or root injuries. The lower roots of the brachial plexus are often subjected to root injuries. The severe lumbosacral plexus injuries are associated with cauda equina ruptures rather than with root avulsions. Pain is a characteristic and severe condition in the natural history of root ruptures and avulsions, together with loss of motor, sensory, and autonomic functions.

References

Barnett HG, Connolly ES, Lumbosacral nerve root avulsion: report of a case and review of the literature, *J Trauma* **15**:532–535, 1975.

Berthold CH, Carlstedt T, General organization of the transitional region in S1 dorsal rootlets, *Acta Physiol Scand Suppl* **446**:23–42, 1977.

Birch R, Bonney G, Wynn Parry CB, *Surgical Disorders of the Peripheral Nerves*, Churchill Livingstone, London, 1998.

Bonney G, The value of axon responses in determining the site of lesion in traction injuries of the brachial plexus, *Brain* **77**:588–609, 1954.

Carlstedt T, Nerve fibre regeneration across the peripheral–central transitional zone, *J Anat* **190**:51–56, 1997.

Carlstedt T, Anand P, Hallin R *et al.*, Spinal nerve root repair and reimplantation of avulsed ventral roots into the spinal cord after brachial plexus injury, *J Neurosurg* **93**:237–247, 2000.

Carlstedt T, Grane P, Hallin R, Noren G, Return of function after spinal cord implantation of avulsed spinal nerve roots, *Lancet* **346**:1323–1325, 1995.

Carlstedt T, Noren G, Repair of ruptured spinal nerve roots in a brachial plexus lesion, *J Neurosurg* **82**:661–663, 1995.

Carvalho GA, Nikkah G, Matties C *et al.*, Diagnosis of root avulsion in traumatic brachial plexus injuries. The value of computerized tomography, myelography and magnetic resonance imaging, *J Neurosurg* **86**:69–76, 1997.

Cilluffo JM, Miller RH, Posttraumatic arachnoid diverticula, *Acta Neurochir* **54**:77–87, 1980.

Cohen-Gadol AA, Krauss WE, Spinner RJ, Delayed central nervous system superficial siderosis following brachial plexus avulsion injury, *Neurosurg Focus* **16**: article 10, 2004.

DaSilva VR, Al-Gahtany M, Midha R *et al.*, Upper thoracic spinal cord herniation after traumatic nerve root avulsion, *J Neurosurg* **99**:306–309, 2003.

Delmas PF, Roger B, Travers V *et al.*, L'exploration moderne des traumatismes du plexus lombo-ischiatique, *J Radiol* **67**:115–118, 1986.

Eisenberg KS, Shift DJ, Murray WR, Posterior dislocation of the hip producing lumbosacral nerve root avulsion. A case report, *J Bone Joint Surg [Am]* **54**:1083–1086, 1972.

Finney LA, Wulfman WA, Traumatic intradural lumbar nerve root avulsion with associated traction injury to the common peroneal nerve, *Am J Roentgenol Radium Ther Nucl Med* **84**:952–957, 1960.

Goodell CL, Neurological deficits associated with pelvic fractures, *J Neurosurg* **24**:837–842, 1966.

Haftek J, Strech injury of peripheral nerve. Acute effects of stretching on a rabbit nerve, *J Bone Joint Surg* **52**:534–565, 1970.

Harris WB, Rathbun JB, Wortzman G, Humphrey JG, Avulsion of lumbar roots complicating fracture of the pelvis, *J Bone Joint Surg* **55**:1436–1442, 1973.

Huittinen VM, Lumbosacral nerve injury in fracture of the pelvis, A post-mortem radiographic and pathoanatomical study, *Acta Chir Scand Suppl* **429**:7–43, 1972.

Huittinen VM, Slätis P, Nerve injury in double vertical pelvic fractures, *Acta Chir Scand* **138**:571–575, 1971.

Kline DG, Donner TR, Happel L *et al.*, Intraforaminal repair of plexus spinal nerves by a posterior approach: an experimental study, *J Neurosurg* **76**:459–470, 1992.

Koliatsos VE, Price WL, Prado CA, Price DL, Ventral root avulsion: an experimental model of death of adult motor neurons, *J Comp Neurol* **342**:35–44, 1994.

Livesey FJ, Fraher JP, Experimental traction injury of the cervical spinal nerve roots: a scanning EM study of rupture pattern in fresh tissue, *Neuropathol Appl Neurobiol* **18**:376–386, 1992.

Mansat M, Anatomie topographique chirurgicale du plexus brachial, *Rev Chir Orthop Reparatrice Appar Mot* **63**:20–26, 1977.

Mansat M, Lebarbier P, Mansat A, Mécanismes lésionnels dans les traumatismes fermés du plexus brachial, in Michon J, Moberg E (eds.), *Lésions traumatiques des nerfs périphériques*, Expansion Scientifique Française, Paris, France, pp. 159–164, 1979.

Moschilla G, Song S, Chakera T, Post-traumatic nerve root avulsion, *Australas Radiol* **45**:281–284, 2001.

Narakas AO, Lesions found when operating traction injuries of the brachial plexus, *Clin Neurol Neurosurg* **95**(Suppl):56–64, 1993.

Penfield W, Late spinal paralysis after avulsion of the brachial plexus, *J Bone Joint Surg* **31**:40–41, 1949.

Privat JM, Mailhe D, Bonnel F, Hémilaminectomie cervicale exploratrice et neurotisation précoce du plexus brachial, *Neurochirurgie* **28**:107–113, 1982.

Stoehr M, Traumatic and postoperative lesions of the lumbosacral plexus, *Arch Neurol* **35**:757–760, 1978.

Sunderland S, Mechanism of cervical nerve root avulsion in injuries of the neck and shoulder, *J Neurosurg* **41**:705–714, 1974.

Sunderland S, Bradley KC, Stress–strain phenomena in human spinal nerve roots, *Brain* **84**:120–124, 1961.

Walter H, Fairholm D, Giant intraspinal pseudomeningoceles cause delayed neurological dysfunction after brachial plexus injury: report of three cases, *Neurosurg* **46**:1245–1249, 2000.

Wynn Parry CB, Pain in avulsion lesions of the brachial plexus, *Pain* **9**:41–53, 1980.

Zorub DS, Nashold BS, Cook WA, Avulsion of the brachial plexus: part I. A review with the implications on the therapy of intractable pain, *Surg Neurol* **2**:347–353, 1974.

3

SURGICAL ANATOMY

Spinal nerve root lesion is considered a type of central nervous injury, and hence is not amenable to operative repair (Seddon 1972). However, it is an anatomical fact that the spinal nerve roots are the intraspinal parts of the peripheral nervous system (PNS) that connect the spinal cord with the peripheral nerves. Regeneration of injured nerve fibres is therefore possible in the spinal nerve roots (Cajal 1928).

The Brachial Plexus (Fig. 1)

The general concept is that the brachial plexus originates from the spinal nerves C5–C8 and T1. In some cases, there might be contributions from neighbouring roots C4 (prefixed plexus) or T2 (postfixed plexus) (von Lanz and Wachsmuth 1955). Outside the intervertebral foramen, there are quite frequent communications between C4 and C5 spinal nerves, as well as branches to the phrenic nerve from C5 and occasionally also from C6. Inside the spinal canal, communications between different roots can occur. This has been described for the dorsal roots C4 to C7. Communicating fibres usually connect to the next rostral root (Perneczky and Sunder-Plassmann 1980). Less frequently, there are also anastomoses between ventral roots (Benini 1987). These variations in anatomy obviously reflect individual differences in dermatomes and myotomes with regards to the distribution of spinal cord segments and spinal roots, as they have been

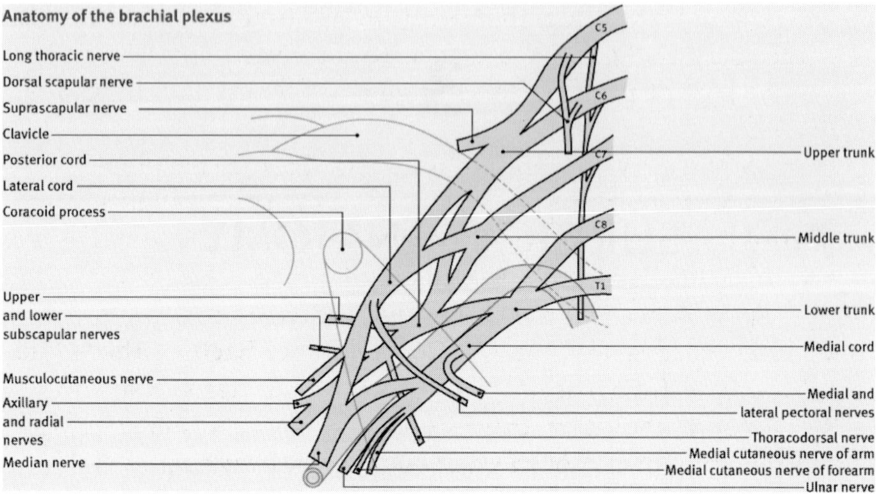

Fig. 1 Schematic drawing of the brachial plexus (from Mannan, Carlstedt, *Surgery* **24**:409–414, 2006).

reported in a variety of pathological conditions causing cervical root compression (Benini 1987) as well as experimentally (Slipman *et al.* 1998). During a proper and complete surgical brachial plexus exploration, these anatomical variations become obvious. The main cause of individual variation in the patterns of innervation is, however, the significant interconnections along the brachial plexus.

Generally, the C5 spinal nerve is responsible for shoulder control and movements as well as for sensation at the shoulder down to the elbow. The C6 spinal nerve usually innervates elbow flexors, including the brachioradial muscle, the supinator and pronator muscles, as well as the extensor carpi radialis longus and the flexor carpi radialis. This nerve also gives sensation in the hand to the thumb and index fingers. The C7 spinal nerve has a diffuse area of innervation in the brachial plexus, jointly with other spinal nerves. It certainly innervates the latissimus dorsi muscle and is responsible — together with other spinal nerves — for elbow extension, wrist extension, finger flexion (flexor digitorum superficialis), and innervation of the middle part of the hand and the fingers. The C8 spinal nerve innervates the extensors and flexors of the fingers and wrist together with the C7 and T1 spinal nerves. The intrinsics of the hand are mainly innervated by C8 and T1. The ulnar part of the hand and fingers are innervated by C8, but not by T1.

Outside the intervertebral foramen, the C5 and C6 spinal nerves have a marked downward course; whereas the C7 has a less downward direction, running almost parallel to C8. The T1 spinal nerve, on the other hand, ascends in a distal direction. The C5–C7 spinal nerves are attached by the transverse radicular ligaments to the transverse processes of the C4–C6 vertebrae. Each of these ligaments extends from the lateral border of the transverse process of the vertebra above or rostral to each nerve, and attaches laterally to the epineurium of the nerves (Fig. 2) (Herzberg *et al.* 1996). This is a unique arrangement; nowhere else along the neuraxis are the nerve roots so firmly anchored to the spine. This certainly offers protection against traction strain to this part of the brachial plexus.

The lower intervertebral foramina are bigger (about 5 × 8 mm) than the more rostral C5 and C6 (4 × 7 mm). The spinal nerves are usually situated in the centre of the foramina, where they each occupy about 50% of the space. The residual space is filled with loose connective tissue. Except for the C5–C7 spinal nerve roots, the nerve roots are only weakly fixated to the wall of the foramen by means of some exchange of connective tissue from the dura investing the nerve roots with the capsule of the facet joint.

The Lumbosacral Plexus and Cauda Equina (Fig. 3)

The lumbar plexus forms from the L1–L4 ventral rami, with a contribution from T12. The sacral plexus derives from the S1–S3 ventral rami, with a contribution from S4 and most importantly from the lumbosacral trunk originating out of the L4 and L5 spinal nerves. There are several intradural and extradural anastomoses described (Chotigavanich and Swangnatra 1992; Kadish and Simmons 1984; Postacchini *et al.* 1982). The main nerves in the lumber plexus are the femoral nerve (L1–L4) and the obturator nerve (L2–L4); and in the

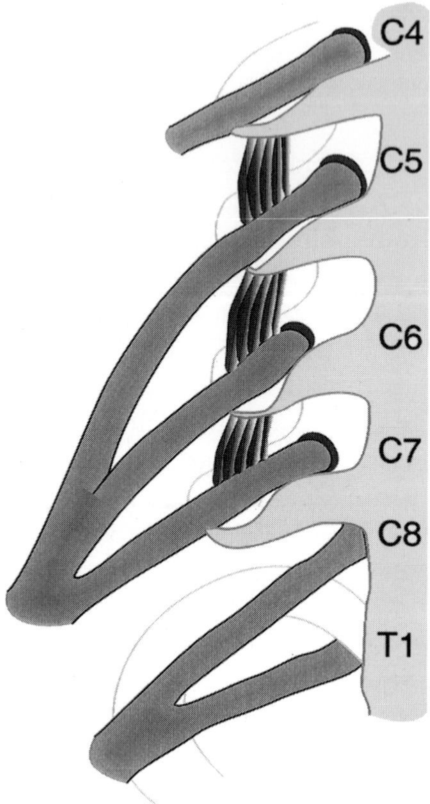

Fig. 2 Attachment of brachial plexus spinal nerves to the cervical spine.

sacral plexus, the sciatic nerve (L4–S3) and the superior gluteal nerve (L4–S1), which innervate the gluteus medius and minimus muscles, and the inferior gluteal nerve (L5–S2) which supplies the gluteus maximus muscle. The posterior femoral cutaneous nerve (S1–S3) is also of diagnostic importance (see below). There are large variations in the standard pattern of innervation from the lumbosacral plexus, but the innervation from the first two sacral nerves to the gastrocnemius muscle is rather constant. S2 also innervates the glutei and the biceps femoris, whereas S3 usually innervates the toe flexors but rarely any other muscles in the limb. S4 does not innervate any limb muscles (Brindley 1994).

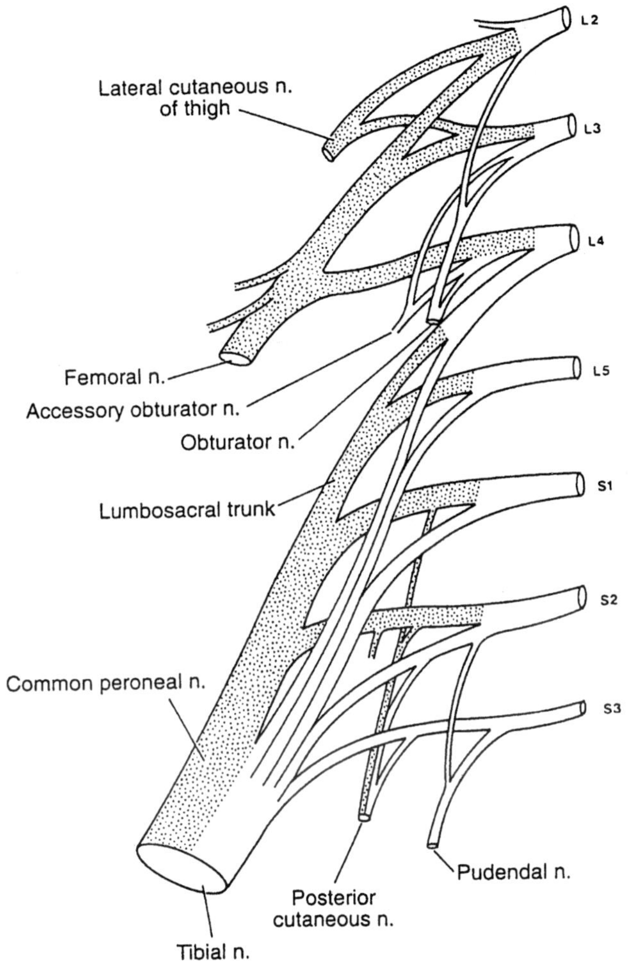

Fig. 3 Schematic drawing of the human lumbosacral plexus. Reproduced from Birch R, Bonney G, Wynn Parry CB, *Surgical Disorders of the Peripheral Nerves*, Churchill Livingstone, Edinburgh, Scotland, 1998, with permission from Dr R. Birch.

The Root Sheath

At the intervertebral canal, the roots are surrounded by an extension of the dura sac forming the root pouch. This ends distally, where the two roots pass distally through separate openings or ostia into the root sleeves (Fig. 4). The dura and the arachnoid invaginate each of

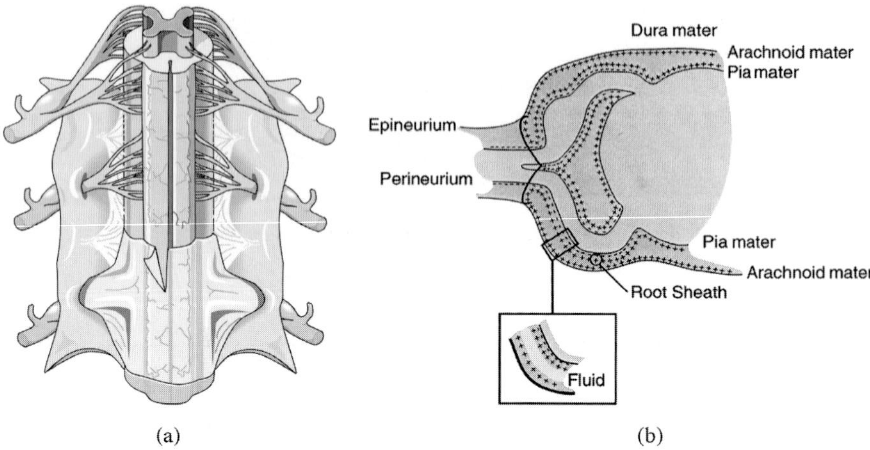

Fig. 4 (a) Schematic drawing of meninges and root sheath. (b) Details of the meninges in the root sheath.

the dorsal and ventral roots, forming two individual sleeves (Mansat 1977). At the root ostia, the subarachnoid fluid is prevented from entering the root sleeve by an adhesion of the arachnoid (Fig. 4). The two roots join distal to the dorsal root ganglion to form the spinal nerve. It is therefore possible during dissection to separate the two roots from each other up to the most distal point of the dorsal root ganglion. The ventral root is here situated caudal (below) rather than ventral to the dorsal root. The meninges continue along the spinal nerve and form a strong epineural sheath.

Within the spinal canal, the roots traverse the subarachnoid space surrounded by a root sheath and bathed in cerebrospinal fluid (CSF). The root sheath consists of an outer layer that resembles the arachnoid and an inner layer that resembles the perineurium (Haller and Low 1971). The outer layer consists of loosely arranged cells with intervening spaces, a pattern reflected back on to the arachnoid in the subarachnoid angle at the distal end of the root. At the root–spinal cord junction or dorsal root entry zone (DREZ), this layer is continuous with the pia mater (Nabeshima *et al.* 1975). The inner layer consists of flattened cells closely associated with an overlaying basal lamina. This layer is continuous with the perineurium distally and terminates close to the root–spinal cord junction proximally, being open-ended towards the spinal cord. Most of the perineurium surrounding the spinal nerve separates from the nerve and continues along the inner surface of the dura mater, as does all of the epineurium (Fig. 4) (Pease and Schultz 1958).

These anatomical conditions have direct practical clinical consequences, as the frail root sheath offers little protection to the root nerve fibres against chemical or mechanical strain. It does not preserve from traction and is not suitable for use in suturing stumps of a severed root together. The barrier function of the perineurium is not present in the root sheath. The chemical environment of the nerve fibres in the root is directly exposed and influenced by the composition of the cerebrospinal fluid (Rydevik *et al.* 1990).

Blood Supply

The vessels of the proximal brachial plexus with topographic relationships have been thoroughly described (Herzberg *et al.* 1996). The ascending cervical artery, which is a branch from the thyrocervical trunk off the subclavian artery, supplies the origin of the upper spinal nerves C5–C7. The lower nerves C8 and T1 are supplied by numerous vessels, such as the intercostal arteries from the costocervical trunk, that follow the course of the T1 and C8 spinal nerves into their foramina. The vertebral arteries bring most of the blood to the cervical spinal cord and its roots. This is of obvious clinical relevance, particularly if during the trauma the subclavian artery has sustained a traction injury from dislocation of the forequarter or if fractures of transverse processes have interrupted circulation in the vertebral artery. Such injuries to the major vessels in the neck could well lead to an infarct in the pertinent spinal cord segment with deterioration of function and neuronal loss (see Chap. 2).

The spinal nerve roots and pertinent spinal cord segments are supplied by a collateral vascular system that derives from two sets of arteries (Fig. 5): the proximal radicular arteries, arising from the medullary artery situated on the spinal cord surface; and the distal radicular arteries, which are branches of the spinal or segmental

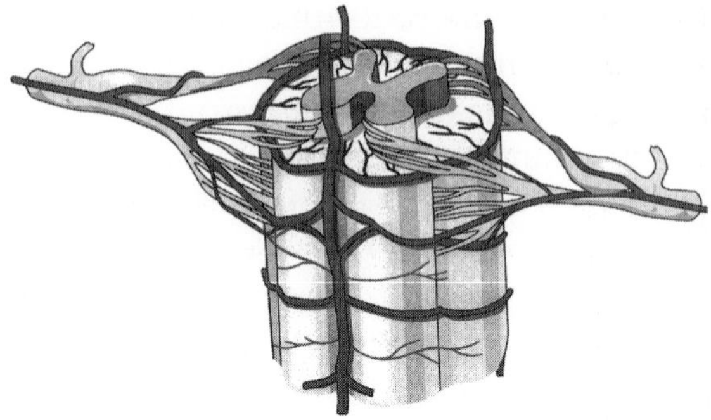

Fig. 5 The collateral vascular system for roots and spinal cord: proximal radicular arteries, arising from the medullary artery situated on the spinal cord surface; and distal radicular arteries, which are branches of the spinal or segmental arteries situated outside the spine.

arteries situated outside the spine. The capillaries from those vessels in the root are of the continuous type, as in the peripheral nerve. They are able to maintain a blood–nerve or blood–root barrier (Yoshizawa *et al.* 1991; Kobayashi *et al.* 1993). In contrast to the peripheral nerve, there are no lymphatic vessels in the root.

Generally, the collateral vascular supply of roots and spinal cord segments guarantees a persistent blood supply, but unfortunately there are inconsistencies among those vessels, particularly for the lower cervical anterior radicular arteries (Turnbull *et al.* 1966). The patency of this collateral vascular system can therefore be dubious. In fact, there is no "safe" area from collaterals of the root or spinal cord circulation. The medullary artery is not always able to maintain adequate circulation in a pertinent root or spinal cord segment if the extraspinal artery has been compromised (Domisse 1975; Park *et al.* 1981), as the anterior spinal artery can be of irregular calibre or even missing (Lazorthes *et al.* 1971). In such cases, the extraspinal vessels may be the only and unique provider of blood supply to the roots and to the pertinent spinal cord segment. Because of the inconsistency of the medullary arteries, the intervertebral foramen is a potential site of origin of a unique feeder vessel to the roots and the spinal cord, and is therefore a vulnerable point in their vascular supply (Domisse 1975).

Severe traction injuries to the brachial plexus with important vascular damage (e.g. proximal rupture of the subclavian or vertebral vessels in conjunction with a brachial plexus injury; see Chap. 2) and multiple root avulsions, where the spinal artery and the roots have been torn, can cause vascular deficit in the pertinent spinal cord segments. In unfortunate cases, vascular insults can present themselves as long tract spinal cord symptoms after a root avulsion injury or after a surgical interference with the local blood supply when operating on the cervical spine. Sometimes, this appears as a Brown–Séquard syndrome. There is an obvious risk of vascular insults to the roots or the spinal cord in conjunction with those injuries. This, of course, should be kept in mind when performing interventions on the cervical spine after root avulsions, and necessary preoperative vascular scanning should be performed (see Chap. 4). Tragic loss of spinal cord function with resulting tetraplegia has happened.

There seems to be larger longitudinal spinal cord vessels and more radicular vascular connections in the lumbosacral region, conferring it great collateral vascular protection. Nevertheless, there is an area of relative hypovascularity in the cauda equina just below the conus medullaris (Park *et al.* 1981). This could have clinical significance in neurogenic claudication concurrent with degenerative changes in the lumbar spine.

The Cervical Nerve Roots

The cervical nerve roots have an oblique course from the intervertebral foramen towards the spinal cord, which they join at an acute angle that is smaller for the T1 than for the C5 root. The rostral roots C5 and C6 (about 15 mm) are shorter than the caudal roots (22–23 mm). The thickness of the roots and the number of rootlets increase from C5 to C7, and then decrease at T1. The distance between the dorsal root entry zone (DREZ) and the ventral root emerging zone (VREZ), i.e. the distance along the spinal cord from the most rostral to the most caudal rootlet junction to the spinal cord, is longer for the more rostral roots compared to the caudal ones (Alleyne *et al.* 1998; Fournier *et al.* 2001). This is of considerable surgical importance, as this is the most frequent site of rupture in brachial plexus avulsion injuries.

At some distance near the spinal cord, the nerve root splits into several rootlets, which in turn separate into still thinner mini-rootlets before joining the spinal cord at the DREZ. The segment situated closest to the DREZ contains a specific and specialized part of the nervous system, where most of the translations between the peripheral nerve and the spinal cord occur (Carlstedt 1977; Fraher 1992; Fraher 2000). This part constitutes the PNS–CNS transitional region (TR) (Fig. 6; see also Chap. 6), which is characterised by the presence of a projection of CNS tissue from the spinal cord together with

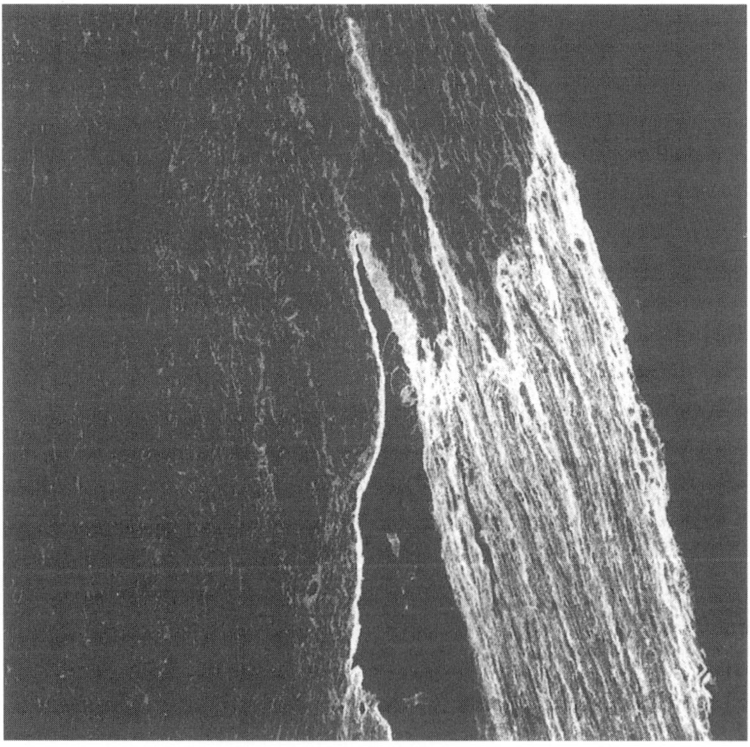

Fig. 6 The proximal part of a rat dorsal root stained for CNS (GFAP) and PNS (laminin) tissue. The protrusion of the spinal cord tissue into the peripheral nerve tissue of the proximal part of the root constitutes the transitional region (from Li *et al.* 2004).

PNS tissue in the most proximal part of the root. The contour of the CNS projection is usually dome-shaped, with a peripherally oriented convexity (Berthold and Carlstedt 1977). The CNS part of the root is longer in dorsal than in ventral roots, and becomes longer in a caudal direction along the spinal cord. The CNS outgrowth is particularly conspicuous in the first sacral root (Tarlov 1937). In cervical ventral roots, where root avulsion is particularly frequent, the PNS–CNS interface is situated beneath the surface of the spinal cord (Fraher 1978). At the PNS–CNS interface, the axon–Schwann cell units cross from the PNS — where they are suspended in an extracellular space containing collagen — into an environment where the extracellular space is exceedingly small, the collagen is lacking, and the axons are embedded in a complex network of oligodendrocyte and astrocyte processes. The vessels of the PNS part of the root do not cross into the CNS.

The interface between the axial CNS tissue in the root and the surrounding PNS tissue is referred to as the CNS–PNS borderline, where nerve fibres extend from the PNS into the CNS and vice versa, traversing the TR. Therefore, this region holds a position of conceptual importance with regard to neuronal organisation, and constitutes a model system for experimental investigations into differences in reaction patterns within one and the same neuron in the peripheral nerve and spinal cord (for details, see Carlstedt *et al.* 2003 and Chap. 6).

The Cervical Spinal Cord

The relation between the cervical spine and the spinal cord is important clinically for orientation on radiographs and scans, as well as intraoperatively. The apex of a cervical vertebra spinous process is usually at the level of the succeeding lower spinal cord segment, e.g. spinal cord segment C7 at the level of the apex of spinous process of C6. When merging to spinal nerves, the roots leave the cervical spine in the intervertebral canal above or rostral to the corresponding vertebra, e.g. C6 spinal nerve leaves the spinal canal in between C5 and C6, but the C6 spinal cord segment is situated at the level of the C5 vertebra. The arrangement of the lower spinal nerves to the brachial plexus is different, as the C8 nerve is situated in the intervertebral canal between vertebrae C7 and T1, and consequently the T1 nerve leaves the spinal canal between vertebrae T1 and T2.

In a cross-section through the cervical spinal cord (Fig. 7), the grey matter is situated around the central canal and extends dorsolaterally as the dorsal horn, or column, almost to the surface of the spinal cord at the posterolateral sulcus. The ventral horn, or column, is shorter and broader than the dorsal horn, and is separated from the spinal cord surface ventrally by about 2 mm and ventrolaterally by about 4 mm (Fournier *et al.* 2001a).

The motor neurons

The motor neurons commanding muscle activity are arranged in longitudinal columns in the ventral horn of the grey matter in the spinal cord. There is a somatotopic arrangement of motoneurons. Those situated in the ventromedial part of the grey matter are innervating

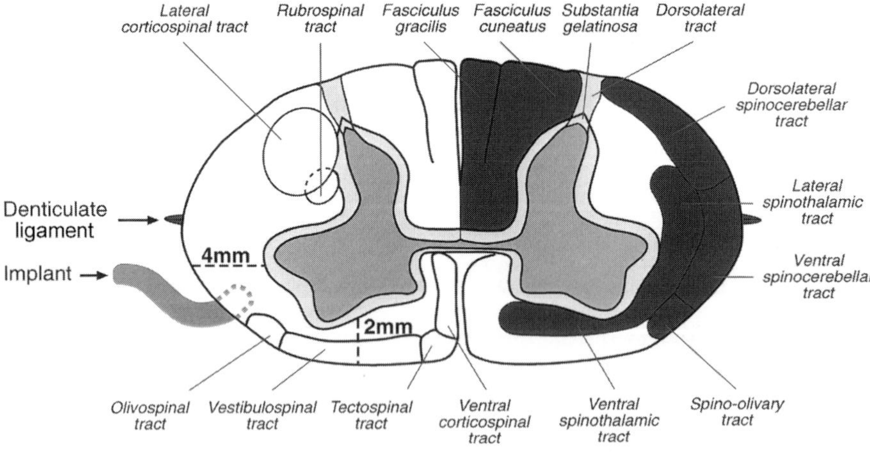

Fig. 7 Schematic drawing of a cross-section through the spinal cord. Descending (motor) tracts are on the left side (white), and ascending (sensory) fibre tracts are on the right side (dark). The distance from surface to motoneuron pool and the preferential site for root or nerve graft implantation is indicated. Modified from Williams PL, Warwick R, Dyson M, Bannister LH (eds.), *Gray's Anatomy*, 37th edn, Churchill Livingstone, London, 1989, with permission from Elsevier Ltd.

trunk muscles, whereas motoneurons in the ventrolateral part innervate muscles distally in the extremity. Extensor muscles are innervated from neurons situated more ventrally than those innervating flexor muscles (Romanes 1946). However, there does not seem to be a specific somatotopic organisation in a particular pool of motoneurons for a specific muscle, but rather in pools innervating functional groups of muscles, e.g. the sciatic motoneuron pool localised in the most lateral and dorsal part of the lumbosacral (L4–S3) ventral horn (Schoenen and Faull 2004). There also seems to be a pattern of overlapping pools for associated muscles. This refers to the arrangement of motoneuron somas; but the sometimes vast dendritic tree, which can extend beyond spinal cord segments, has not been taken into account. An exception is the well-defined phrenic motoneuron pool in the medial part of the ventral horn extending as a column from the C3 to C6 spinal cord segments (Keswani and Hollinshead 1956).

The neurons in the ventral horn of the spinal cord are generally considered in two functional groups as alpha and gamma motoneurons and interneurons. Furthermore, there are fast- and slow-twitch alpha motoneurons innervating striated muscles, while gamma neurons innervate the intrafusal fibres in the muscle spindles for a "servo loop" mechanism of muscle control. The motoneurons mainly connect to dorsal root afferents in the same or neighbouring segment, i.e. monosynaptically to proprioceptic fibres and interneurons, as well as to descending fibre tracts such as the vestibulospinal, tectospinal, reticulospinal, and corticoreticulospinal tracts for axial and medial muscles; rubrospinal tracts for distal muscles; and the corticospinal tracts with which most motoneurons in man make monosynaptic connections (Burke 1990). Acetylcholin is the main neurotransmitter in spinal motoneurons, whereas supraspinal motor systems are served by the major excitatory neurotransmitter glutamate. Calcitonin gene-related peptide (CGRP) is the only peptide identified within the perikarya of motoneurons (Schoenen and Faull 2004).

Trophic factors and receptors of importance to support motoneuron survival and repair are the neurotrophins brain-derived neurotrophic factor (BDNF) and neurotrophin-3; the insulin growth factors (IGFs); and various cytokines such as ciliary neurotrophic factor (CNTF), colinergic differentiation factor/leukaemia inhibitory factor (CDF/LIF), and members of the TGF-beta superfamily (i.e. glia cell line–derived neurotrophic factor or GDNF). In the normal uninjured situation, there are significant levels of BDNF mRNA and mRNA for the IGF receptors ICFR-1 and IGFR-2, but very high mRNA levels for trkB and the GDNF receptors c-RET and GFRa1 (Hammarberg 2000). After injury, particularly ventral root avulsion, there is a dramatic response in molecular production by motoneurons, causing a cascade of subcellular events (see Chap. 6).

The sensory neurons

The primary sensory neurons are located in the dorsal root ganglia (DRG) of the PNS, and project axons both centrally to the spinal cord through the dorsal root transitional region (TR) and the dorsal root entry zone (DREZ) as well as peripherally through the dorsal roots to peripheral targets. The neurons of the DRG are a heterogeneous population in their connectivity and expression of neuropeptides, enzymes, and cell surface antigens. Small- and medium-sized neurons innervate several types of mechanoreceptors, thermoreceptors, and nociceptors in the skin; whereas large neurons innervate proprioceptors. Small DRG neurons react to nerve growth factor (NGF) and GDNF; whereas some intermediate- and large-sized DRG neurons react to BDNF, GDNF, and neurotrophin-3 (NT-3). The neurotrophic factors exert their effects via specific high-affinity binding to receptor tyrosine kinases known as trks: NGF interacts with trkA, BDNF with trkB, and NT-3 with trkC. In addition to their interaction with trk receptors, each neurotrophin is capable of binding to the low-affinity neurotrophin receptor p75. NGF appears to be important in maintaining phenotypic and functional properties in the normal uninjured situation. Almost half of the DRG neurons contain peptides such as CGRP, substance P, galanin, vasoactive intestinal polypeptide (VIP), enkephalin, and somatostatin. Most of these cells are small myelinated and unmyelinated neurons likely to mediate pain, but neuropeptide Y normally occurs in large dorsal root ganglion neurons (McMahon and Priestley 2005).

In the dorsal horn, the two major nucleus columns are the superficially situated substantia gelatinosa, which connects with cutaneous afferents from the dorsal roots and is of importance in pain mechanisms (particularly after root avulsion) (Ovelmen-Levitt 1988), and the deeper nucleus proprius. The finer fibres in the dorsal root related to pain and temperature, which express peptides CGRP and substance P and respond to NGF, terminate in the superficial parts of the dorsal horn (laminae I and II). Larger fibres expressing NPY terminate in deeper parts of the dorsal horn, with proprioceptic fibres ending in the ventral horn at motoneurons. There is a certain somatotopy regarding the arrangement of afferent fibres in the most proximal part of the dorsal root and the dorsal horn. There is a segregation of afferent fibres according to size and function. Large fibres are confined to the centre of the rootlets; whereas small-calibre fibres, which are for instance committed to nociceptive function, are situated at the periphery of the rootlets. More centrally, they are concentrated on the ventral and lateral aspects. In the spinal cord, they will merge with the tract of Lissauer (Carlstedt 1977; Snyder 1977). The specific anatomical arrangement of these fibres is the fundament of selective rhizotomy (Sindou *et al.* 1974). The larger primary sensory fibres from the distal parts of the limb are represented medially, whereas proximal parts of the extremity terminate laterally in the dorsal horn.

The fibre tracts

The main descending fibre tract of importance in humans for motor control is the corticospinal tract. The main part has crossed from contralateral supraspinal origin to become the lateral corticospinal tract. It is situated in the dorsolateral funiculus of the spinal cord, with a near-anatomical relation to the denticulate ligament, particularly in the cervical segments of the spinal cord. A smaller uncrossed part of the corticospinal tract is situated in the anterior funiculus and is known as the ventral corticospinal tract (Nathan *et al.* 1990). In humans, there are roughly one million axons in the corticospinal tract. There are mainly small-diameter fibres, but larger fibres of about 20 μm represent direct cortico-motoneuron connections, which in humans project to the motoneuron groups in the ventral horn for proximal and distal muscle groups (Schoenen and Grant 2004).

In patients subjected to cordotomy for relief of cancer pain, it is known that lesion of the anterior segment of the spinal cord does not lead to paralysis. However, when a cordotomy affects the region posterior to the denticulate ligament or the dorsolateral funiculus, an ipsilateral flaccid paralysis may develop (Nathan 1994). Descending brainstem pathways are also of importance for motor control in humans. These can be divided into two main groups, with different locations and functions. One group (reticulospinal, vestibulospinal, interstitiospinal, and tectospinal tracts) is situated in the ventral and ventrolateral white matter together with the ventral corticospinal fibres (Fig. 7). It is concerned with control of posture, synergistic whole-limb movements, and orientation movements of body and head. The other group (rubrospinal and pontospinal tracts) is situated in the dorsolateral fasciculus together with the crossed or lateral corticospinal tract. These fibres provide control of flexion movements of the extremities, particularly the elbow and the hand. Specifically, the corticospinal tract has been ascribed hand and finger function in the human. As a result, patients with injuries to the corticospinal tract at midcervical level, i.e. at C3–C4, present with severely impaired hand function, such as the inability to button a shirt. This deficit is commonly referred to as a central cord injury.

The ascending tracts are mainly situated in the dorsal columns and the dorsolateral funiculus (Fig. 7). There are current data that these pathways are involved in visceral nociception and highly complex discriminatory tasks such as two-point discrimination (Schoenen and Grant 2004). The spinothalamic tract is situated in the ventrolateral fasciculus, where root reimplantation surgery is performed. This tract originates from contralateral nerve cells. There is good evidence from palliative cordotomies for alleviation of pain (Schoenen 1981) that these fibre tracts are the pathways for pain, temperature, touch, and pressure from the contralateral part of the body (cf. the Brown–Séquard syndrome). In some patients with complete avulsion injury to the brachial plexus, the Brown–Séquard syndrome has developed, probably from interference to spinal cord circulation rather than from direct loss of spinal cord substance in the trauma. A transient postoperative contralateral loss of temperature sensation has occasionally been noted in patients after reimplantation surgery (Carlstedt 1985; Carlstedt *et al.* 2000).

Conclusion

The intraspinal part of the nervous system is mainly of peripheral nervous type, although the spinal nerve roots differ in many respects from a peripheral nerve, mainly with regard to their surrounding sheaths, quality of blood supply, and organisation of nerve fibres. The nerve root contains the interface between the peripheral and central nervous systems, where the same nerve fibres change in their anatomical (but not physiological or chemical) characteristics and in their ability to regrow after injury. In the spinal nerve roots, nerve fibres can regenerate after a nerve injury, just as in the peripheral nervous system.

References

Alleyne CH, Cawley CM, Barrow DL, Bonner GD, Microsurgical anatomy of the dorsal cervical nerve roots and the cervical dorsal root ganglion/ventral root complexes, *Surg Neurol* **50**:213–218, 1998.

Benini A, Clinical features of cervical root compression C5–C8 and their variations, *Neuro-Orthop* **4**:74–88, 1987.

Berthold CH, Carlstedt T, General organization of the transitional region in S1 dorsal rootlets, *Acta Physiol Scand Suppl* **446**:23–42, 1977.

Brindley GS, The first 500 patients with sacral anterior root stimulator implants: general description, *Paraplegia* **32**:795–805, 1994.

Burke RE, Spinal cord: ventral horn, in Shepard GM (ed.), *The Synaptic Organization of the Brain*, Oxford University Press, New York, pp. 88–132, 1990.

Cajal SR, *Degeneration and Regeneration of the Nervous System*, Oxford University Press, London, 1928.

Carlstedt T, Observations on the morphology at the transition between the peripheral and central nervous system in the cat, PhD thesis, Karolinska Institutet, Stockholm, Sweden, 1977.

Carlstedt T, Regenerating axons from nerve terminals at astrocytes, *Brain Res* **347**:188–191, 1985.

Carlstedt T, Anand P, Hallin R *et al.*, Spinal nerve root repair and reimplantation of avulsed ventral roots into spinal cord after brachial plexus injury, *J Neurosurg* **93**:237–247, 2000.

Carlstedt T, Cullheim S, Risling M, Spinal cord in relation to the peripheral system, in Paxinos G, Mai J (eds.), *The Human Nervous System II*, Academic Press, San Diego, CA, pp. 250–263, 2003.

Chotigavanich C, Sawangnatra S, Anomalies of the lumbosacral nerve roots, *Clin Orthop* **278**:46–50, 1992.

Domisse GF, *The Arteries and Veins of the Human Spinal Cord from Birth*, Churchill, Edinburgh, Scotland, 1975.

Fournier HD, Menei P, Khalifa R, Mercier P, Ideal intraspinal implantation site for the repair of ventral root avulsion after brachial plexus injury in humans. A preliminary anatomical study, *Surg Radiol Anat* **23**:191–195, 2001.

Fournier HD, Mercier P, Menei P, Anatomical bases of the posterior approach to the brachial plexus for repairing avulsed spinal nerve roots, *Surg Radiol Anat* **23**:3–8, 2001.

Fraher JP, The maturation of the ventral root–spinal cord transitional zone. An ultrastructural study, *J Neurol Sci* **36**:427–449, 1978.

Fraher JP, The CNS–PNS transitional zone of the rat. Morphometric studies at cranial and spinal levels, *Prog Neurobiol* **38**:261–316, 1992.

Fraher JP, The transitional zone and CNS regeneration, *J Anat* **196**:137–316, 2000.

Haller FR, Low FN, The fine structure of peripheral nerve root sheath in the subarachnoid space in the rat and other laboratory animals, *Am J Anat* **131**:1–20, 1971.

Hammarberg H, Spinal motoneurons and molecules related to neurotrophic function after axon injury, PhD thesis, Karolinska Institutet, Stockholm, Sweden, 2000.

Herzberg G, Narakas A, Comtet J-J, Surgical approach of the brachial plexus roots, in Alnot JY, Narakas A (eds.), *Traumatic Brachial Plexus Injuries*, Expansion Scientifique Française, Paris, France, pp. 19–22, 1996.

Kadish L, Simmons EH, Anomalies of the lumbosacral nerve roots, *J Bone Joint Surg* **66**:411–416, 1984.

Keswani N, Hollinshead WH, Localization of the phrenic nucleus in the spinal cord of man, *Anat Rec* **125**:683–700, 1956.

Kobayashi S, Yoshizawa H, Hachiya Y *et al.*, Vasogenic edema induced by compression injury to the spinal nerve root. Distribution of intravenously injected protein tracers and gadolinium-enhanced magnetic resonance imaging, *Spine* **18**:1410–1424, 1993.

Lazorthes G, Gouaz A, Zadeh JO *et al.*, Arterial vascularization of the spinal cord, *J Neurosurg* **35**:253–262, 1971.

Li Y, Carlstedt T, Berthold CH, Raisman G, Interaction of transplanted olfactory-ensheathing cells and host astrocytic processes provides a bridge for axons to regenerate across the dorsal root entry zone, *Exp Neurol* **188**:300–308, 2004.

Mansat M, Anatomie topographique chirurgicale du plexus brachial, *Rev Chir Orthop Reparatrice Appar Mot* **63**:20–26, 1977.

McMahon SB, Priestley JV, Nociceptor plasticity, in Hunt S, Koltzenburg M (eds.), *The Neurobiology of Pain*, Oxford University Press, Oxford, UK, pp. 35–64, 2005.

Nabeshima S, Reese TS, Landis DMD, Brightman MW, Junction in the meninges and marginal glia, *J Comp Neurol* **164**:127–170, 1975.

Nathan PW, Effects on movements of surgical incisions into the human spinal cord, *Brain* **117**:337–346, 1994.

Nathan PW, Smith MC, Deacon P, The corticospinal tracts in man. Course and location of fibres at different segmental levels, *Brain* **113**:303–324, 1990.

Ovelmen-Levitt J, Abnormal physiology of the dorsal horn as related to the deafferentation syndrome, *Appl Neurophysiol* **51**:104–116, 1988.

Park WW, Gamell K, Rothman RH, Arterial vascularization of the cauda equina, *J Bone Joint Surg [Am]* **63**:53–61, 1981.

Pease DC, Schultz RL, Electron microscopy of rat cranial meninges, *Am J Anat* **102**:301–321, 1958.

Perneczky A, Sunder-Plassmann M, Intradural variant of cervical nerve root fibres. Potential cause of misinterpreting the segmental location of cervical disc prolapses from clinical evidence, *Acta Neurochir (Wien)* **52**:79–83, 1980.

Postacchini F, Urso S, Ferro L, Lumbosacral nerve–root anomalies, *J Bone Joint Surg* **64**:721–729, 1982.

Romanes GJ, Motor localization and the effect of nerve injury on the ventral horn cells of the spinal cord, *J Anat* **80**:117–131, 1946.

Rydevik B, Holm B, Brown MD, Lundborg G, Diffusion from the cerebrospinal fluid as a nutritional pathway for spinal nerve roots, *Acta Physiol Scand* **138**:247–248, 1990.

Schoenen J, *L'organisation Neuronale de la Moelle Épinierè de L'homme*, Editions Sciences et Lettres, Liège, Belgium, 1981.

Schoenen J, Faull RLM, Spinal cord: cyto and chemoarchitecture, in Paxinos G, Mai JK (eds.), *The Human Nervous System II*, Academic Press, San Diego, CA, pp. 190–232, 2004.

Schoenen J, Grant G, Spinal cord: connections, in Paxinos G, Mai JK (eds.), *The Human Nervous System II*, Academic Press, San Diego, CA, pp. 233–249, 2004.

Seddon HF, *Surgical Disorders of the Peripheral Nerves*, Williams and Wilkins, Baltimore, MD, 1972.

Sindou M, Quoex C, Baleydier C, Fiber organization at the posterior spinal cord–rootlet junction in man, *J Comp Neurol* **153**:15–26, 1974.

Slipman CW, Plastaras CT, Palmitier RA *et al.*, Symptom provocation of fluoroscopically guided cervical nerve root stimulation, *Spine* **23**:2235–2242, 1998.

Snyder R, The organization of the dorsal root entry zone in cats and monkeys, *J Comp Neurol* **174**:47–56, 1977.

Tarlov IM, Structure of the nerve root. I. Nature of the junction between the central and the peripheral nervous system, *Arch Neurol Psychiatr* **37**:555, 1937.

Turnbull IM, Brieg A, Hassler O, Blood supply of cervical spinal cord in man, *J Neurosurg* **24**:951–965, 1966.

Von Lantz T, Wachsmuth W, *Praktische Anatomie: Ein Lehr-und Hilfsbuch der anatomischen Grundlagen ärzlichen Handelns*, Springer-Verlag, Berlin, pp. 27–29, 1955.

Yoshizawa H, Kobayashi S, Hachiya Y, Blood supply of nerve roots and dorsal root ganglia, *Orthop Clin North Am* **22**:195–211, 1991.

4

ASSESSMENT OF PATIENTS WITH INTRASPINAL PLEXUS INJURIES

Clinical Examination

The brachial plexus

A carefully taken history, together with a clinical examination based on neuroanatomy (see Chap. 3), often gives a good indication of total or partial brachial plexus avulsion. This applies to an early assessment of the patient, as the intraspinal plexus lesion can only be operated within a narrow time-window to be successful.

History. It is important to learn about the mechanism and violence of the trauma. A typical history of severe intraspinal brachial plexus injury is seen in patients involved in motorcycle accidents. For instance, they may show a displacement of the forequarter, their shoulder having struck against a traffic bollard. These lesions are usually thought of as injuries of high-speed accidents, but there are cases of complete avulsion injury in motorcyclists whose speed at the time of accident was less than 50 km/h and even in pedal cyclists. The "classical" cause originally described in the eighth book of Homer's *Iliad* (Robotti *et al.* 1995), namely a stone or boulder falling onto the shoulder, is also seen in various other traumas. It is obviously the magnitude of the force hitting the forequarter that is of importance and should, if possible, be appreciated during the assessment.

In cases of root avulsion, the patient is often able to describe the typical root avulsion pain. This is perceived in most patients immediately after the trauma as a constant dull, crushing, or burning pain with superimposed lightning jolts of severe sharp pain shooting down the arm. In at least half of the patients, this pain can be felt immediately after the accident, but can also start some days later. The first case of complete brachial plexus avulsion injury that was explored in 1911 by Frazier and Skillern was sustained by a physician who had been injured when, walking along a street, he was hit by a man falling from the fourth floor of a building. He gave the following description of his pain: "The pain is continuous; it does not stop a minute either day or night. It is either burning or compressing (like a vice) or dragging (a sense of weight) in character, or a combination of all these at the same time. Every few minutes this pain is intensified in a paroxysm lasting from a few seconds to a minute or longer [...] I have a graphic picture of it in my mind; it is like zigzag made in the skies by a stroke of lightning. The pain is felt sometimes in the very arm itself, but most of the time away from the arm, in what I got into the habit of calling an imaginary arm. The upper part of the arm is mostly free from pain; the lower part from a little above the elbow to the tips of the fingers, never. Pain of every character, burning, compressing, dragging or jerking is increased by walking, standing or even sitting up, so that the recumbent position is a necessity for most of the day" (cited in Frazier and Skillern 1911).

It is, of course, important to know about the patient's general health and to carefully investigate medications. For instance, the use of aspirin is contraindicated with spinal cord surgery.

Inspection. A Bernard–Horner sign indicates, but is not absolute proof of, avulsion of the lower roots of the plexus. This sign may not be obvious immediately after the accident. Bruising and swelling at the base of the neck are important and sometimes ominous signs (Fig. 1). Abrasions can appear as linear cuts passing from the face towards the shoulder, indicating a violent distraction of the limb

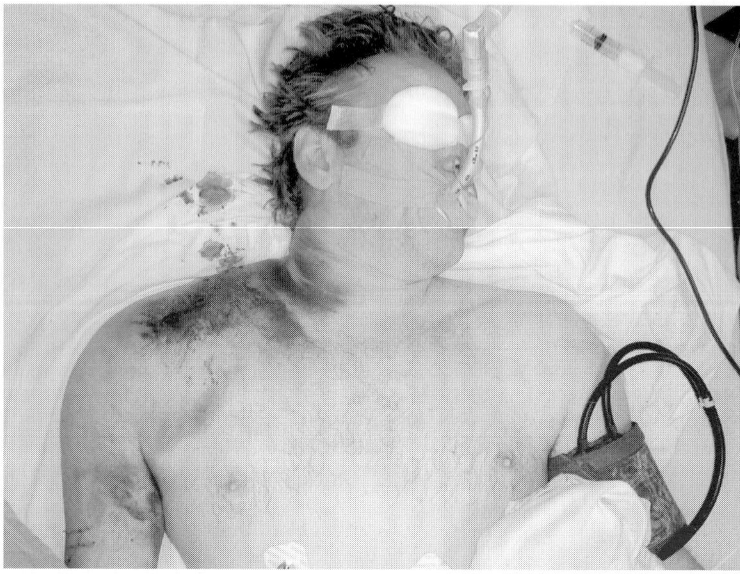

Fig. 1 Severe trauma to the shoulder and the base of the neck in a road traffic accident. Haematoma and swelling indicate a lesion of the longitudinal neurovascular structures.

from the neck. There could be tears of the muscles at the base of the neck, a collection of cerebrospinal fluid from root avulsions, or even rupture of large vessels, particularly if the swelling is expanding. If the distal pulse is missing, an angiography is necessary; and if an abolition of flow in the subclavian or axillary artery is diagnosed (Fig. 2), the patient needs urgent vascular reconstruction notwithstanding the perfusion of the limb through collateral vessels.

Examination. The brachial plexus, if *in situ*, can be palpated as a ridge just lateral to the sternocleidomastoid muscle. If this is not felt, the plexus may have been pulled underneath the clavicle. Tapping on the site of the plexus can elicit a sharp electric sensation shooting down the arm. This is Tinel's sign: a reliable sign indicating that there is at least one spinal nerve ruptured outside the spinal canal, which could be used for extraspinal repair. This sign can be provoked early, at least within days after the injury, and gives a painful sensation of paraestesia radiating down to the elbow for a

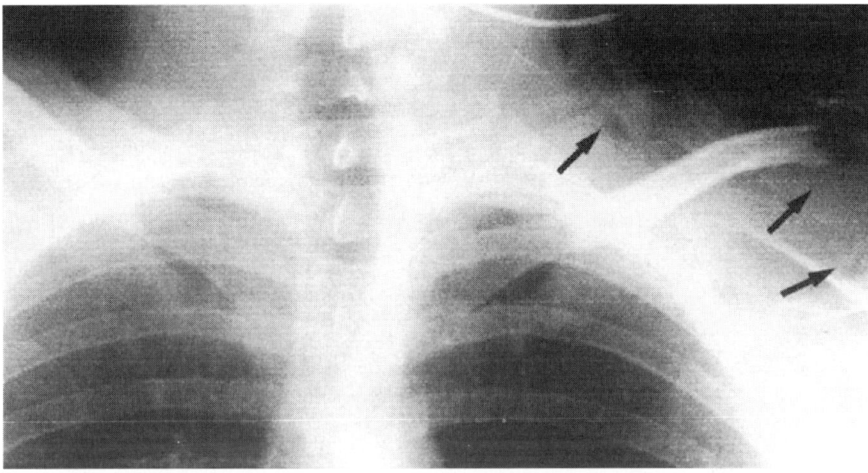

(a)

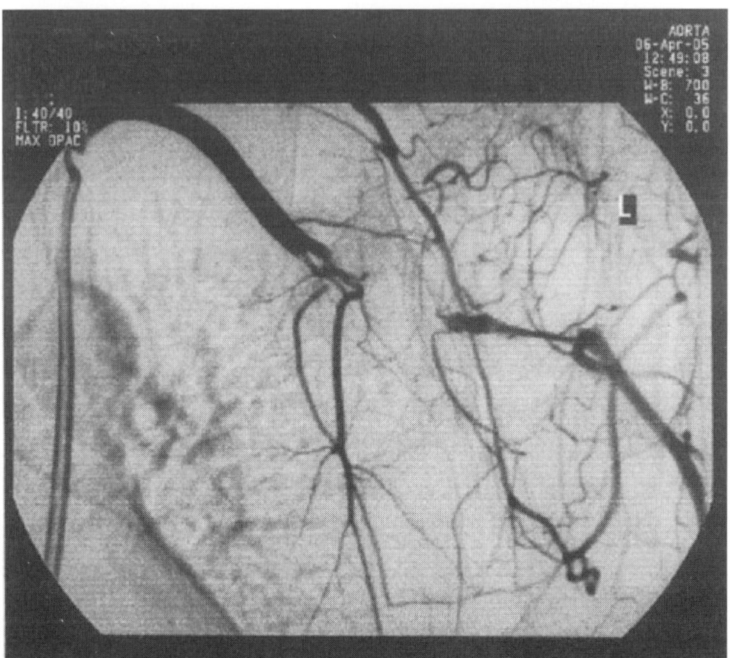

(b)

Fig. 2 A case of traumatic scapula thorax dissociation. (a) The forequarter was severely displaced during the impact, resulting in fractures of the scapula and clavicula together with soft tissue injuries (arrows). (b) Angiography revealed an intima lesion of the axillary artery that has blocked blood flow, but there is collateral circulation. An arterial repair is necessary together with plexus reconstruction.

C5 stump, to the radial part of the hand for C6, and to the back of the hand for C7.

If no Tinel's sign can be provoked in a patient with complete paralysis, but a Bernard–Horner sign and typical avulsion pain are present, the clinical assessment points towards a rather complete avulsion of all five spinal nerves of the brachial plexus. This in itself is a spinal cord lesion that affects the local segmental spinal cord circuits for the arm. Besides, some of these patients also have signs of compromised long fibre tract function, i.e. the Brown–Séquard syndrome. This is more likely to be the effect of the interruption of radicular vascular supply to the spinal cord rather than a direct medullary trauma.

Muscle testing. This is a truncated description of the method for muscle testing in the upper extremity as taught to registrars. What follows is relevant for an assessment of what appears to be a complete brachial plexus injury possibly with avulsions, where invasive examinations like myelography and CT scanning are considered, followed by intraspinal repair. For a full description of testing for muscle function, see Seddon (1954).

Spared function indicates one or more spinal root ruptures. For example, activity in the serratus anterior muscle only could mean that there are one or more proximal stumps of spinal nerves C5–C7. A positive Tinel's sign supports the possibility of proximal stumps from spinal nerve rupture. However, it is not uncommon that the roots have been avulsed, but some fascicles for the long thoracic nerve have been spared and are still in continuity with the spinal cord, although the plexus (with roots and ganglia) is found detached from the intervertebral foramina during exploration.

Activity in the supraspinatus muscle innervated by the suprascapular nerve, which is the next nerve distal to the long thoracic nerve, reveals a longer proximal stump including not only C5 but possibly also C6, i.e. a rupture at the level of the upper trunk. This is a very good sign, making an exclusive extraspinal repair possible. With activity also in the clavicular part of the pectoral muscle, integrity of the upper part of the brachial plexus with a rupture at the clavicular level is revealed.

Function in the sternal part of the pectoral muscle shows that the lower part of the brachial plexus, formed by the C8 and T1 spinal nerves, is intact, and function should be expected in the muscles of the hand and below the elbow. In cases with a distal rupture of the upper part of the brachial plexus and/or a lesion in the continuity of the lower trunk of the brachial plexus, intraspinal repair should not be considered but rather repair of the nerves, supplemented if needed by nerve transfers (see Chap. 7).

When performing the assessment, one should start from the top and ask the patient to shrug his shoulders to test the power in the trapezius muscle. Of course, this muscle is not innervated by the brachial plexus, but the accessory nerve is useful for transfer into the plexus, particularly for the suprascapular nerve. Therefore, it needs to be tested (see Chap. 5).

Next comes the test of the serratus anterior, which is innervated by the long thoracic nerve. This nerve is the first to leave the plexus at the outer mouth of the intervertebral canal. It must be remembered that activity in the serratus muscle does not preclude avulsion. As the patient cannot lift his arm to press against the wall, which is the classical way of testing this muscle on isolated palsy, the arm should be supported by the assessor and the patient asked to push forwards as if trying to open a door (Fig. 3). At the same time, the examiner should hold the apex or the lower pool of the scapula in between the thumb and the index finger. Any activity in the serratus anterior will be revealed by the movements of the apex of the scapula.

The rhomboids should also be checked by asking the patient to brace the shoulder blades. There is usually function, as these muscles are innervated from outside the plexus by the dorsal scapula nerve, which can be used for transfer.

The pectoral muscle is really a key muscle in telling if there is an upper, lower, or total proximal lesion. Asking the patient to try to touch his contralateral shoulder across his chest, or supporting him in doing so, would reveal function in the clavicular part of the pectoral muscle, innervated from the upper part of the plexus (C5–C7) through the lateral pectoral nerve [Fig. 4; see also Chap. 8, Fig. 1(a)]. Asking the patient to adduct his arm towards the side of his chest,

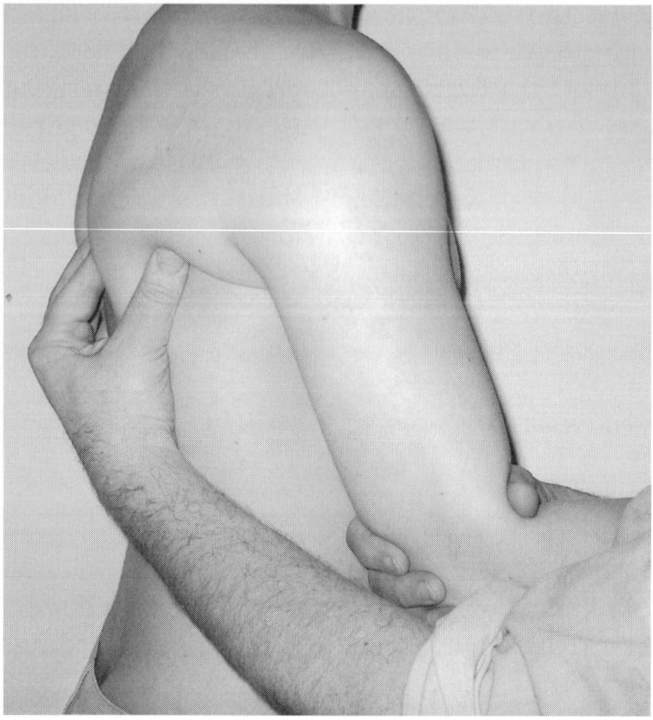

Fig. 3 Test of serratus anterior function in cases of global arm palsy. The apex of the scapula is pinched between the thumb and the index fingers. Movements of the scapula when the patient is trying to press his arm forwards reveals long thoracic nerve function.

as if holding a newspaper under the arm, reveals the power of the sternal part of this muscle, innervated from the lower part of the plexus (C8–T1) through the medial pectoral nerve (Fig. 4).

The rotator cuff muscles, supraspinatus, and infraspinatus are innervated mainly from C5 through the suprascapular nerve. Activity in the supraspinatus is difficult to feel underneath the trapezius, but function is of course revealed by the initiation of abduction. The infraspinatus can be felt lateral to the trapezius. If strong enough, it allows external rotation; but again, the elbow might need support as there could be a paralysis of elbow flexion.

Elbow flexion and extension are rather straightforward tests. Flexion is mainly innervated by C6, but there are wide variations.

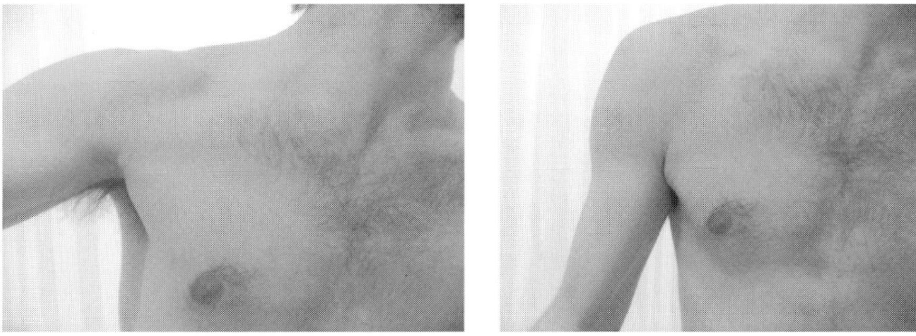

(a) (b)

Fig. 4 Activity in the pectoral muscle indicates the integrity of (a) the upper part of the plexus for the clavicular part and (b) the lower part of the plexus for the sternal part.

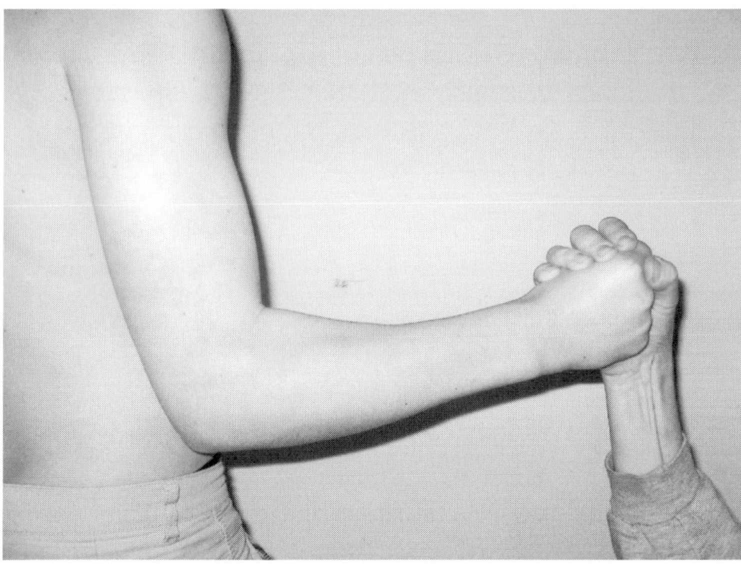

Fig. 5 The brachioradial muscle can act as a powerful elbow flexor and mask palsy caused by musculocutaneous nerve impairment.

One should be aware that the powerful brachioradial muscle can perform an excellent elbow flexion on its own (Fig. 5). The contractions in the biceps and the brachial muscles must be palpated. It is also easy to assess elbow extension allowed by the triceps, the three heads of which are innervated by C5–C7, sometimes even by the lower spinal nerves C8 and T1.

Forearm and wrist movements, i.e. prosupination, wrist flexion (FCR), and wrist extension (ECRL), are generally made possible by the C6 nerve.

Hand function is mainly innervated by the lower spinal nerves of the plexus, C8, and T1. Intrinsic function is tested by thumb–index finger pinch (Froment's test) and abduction–opposition of the thumb. In cases of extensor digitorum communis palsy, abduction and adduction of the fingers can be assessed by supporting the patient's hand in the palm and asking him to spread his fingers (Fig. 6). However, extension of IP joints in the fingers should not be confused with weak EDC function. Sensation in the hand is due to C6 for the radial part, C7 for the middle part, and C8 for the ulnar part of the hand.

In cases of subtotal brachial plexus lesion with some spared hand function, it should be considered that a single spinal nerve such as C7, C8, or T1 is still in continuity. Good sensation in the ulnar

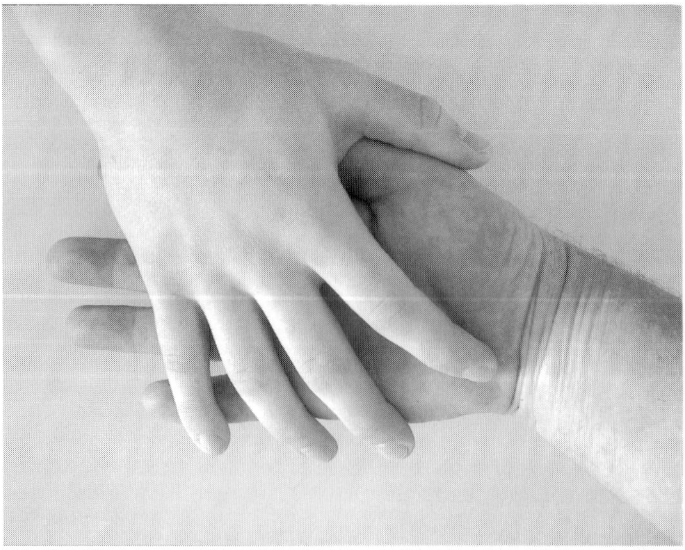

Fig. 6 Intrinsic function tested when there is extensor paralysis.

fingers with intrinsic function indicates a spared C8. A patchy sensory perception in the hand with mainly thenar muscle function could mean that C7 alone is partly active. If the patient shows a complete loss of sensation in the hand, but some muscle function is present, T1 alone is still functioning. In such cases, when only one of the lower spinal nerves of the plexus has been spared, nerve transfers to recover elbow function, for instance from the ulnar nerve, are dubious with small chances of useful recovery.

The lumbosacral plexus

Clinical diagnosis of the level of an injury in the lumbosacral plexus is much more difficult than in cases of brachial plexus lesions. The lumbosacral plexus, confined deep within the pelvis, cannot be assessed by means of palpation or by tapping to provoke a Tinel's sign. Moreover, few nerve branches stem from its proximal part, making an appreciation of the type of injury depending on spared activity, i.e. intraspinal in the cauda equina or intrapelvic, quite difficult. However, there are two useful nerves in this respect: the superior gluteal nerve, which arises from the L5 nerve or lumbosacral trunk, as well as from the S1 spinal nerve in the proximal part of the lumbosacral plexus; and the posterior cutaneous nerve of the thigh, which is formed at the lateral part of the sacral plexus as the sacral spinal nerves merge to form the sciatic nerve. When activity in the gluteus medius muscle, innervated by the superior gluteal nerve, is the only function present in the leg, this indicates an intrapelvic rather than a cauda equina lesion. As for the posterior cutaneous nerve of the thigh, loss of function in the hamstring muscles and in all muscles distal to the knee, with pelvic stability (negative Trendelenburg test) and sensation on the back of the thigh, points to a high sciatic rather than a sacral plexus injury.

Ancillary Investigations

Electrophysiology

Initially, within days after the injury, electrophysiological assessment of the plexus injury is of little value. Stimulation of a severed nerve distal to the lesion can still give rise to muscle contractions up to 2–3 days after the injury. It is only 2 to 3 weeks after the injury that the typical denervation signs, i.e. positive sharp waves and fibrillations, become obvious, once the Wallerian degeneration has interfered with the trophic support of the motor nerves to the muscles (Weddell *et al.* 1944). Although the severity of the nerve injury (neurotmesis or axonotmesis) is difficult to appreciate with electrophysiology, the less serious neuropraxia lesion can be revealed by means of the presence of a compound action potential.

The presence of a sensory nerve action potential (SNAP), together with loss of sensation in the distribution for a particular nerve, is an ominous sign of a root lesion. After such a proximal lesion, the spinal root ganglion will still be active and its nerve cells can support nerve action potentials distally; but, as there is no connection centrally to the spinal cord, there is no perception of the sensory stimulus (Fig. 7). Stimulation of sensation distally for the different spinal cord segments should be a simple investigation. Recordings of sensory action potentials indicate an injury proximal to the ganglion. This test is reliable if performed after Wallerian degeneration is completed, but can give confusing results if performed earlier. However, even if performed correctly, it is not useful in cases of severe complete brachial plexus avulsion, as surgery should not be delayed and certainly not for the sake of investigations. Together with clinical signs such as the absence of a Tinel's sign, the presence of Horner's syndrome, and complete motor and sensory loss,

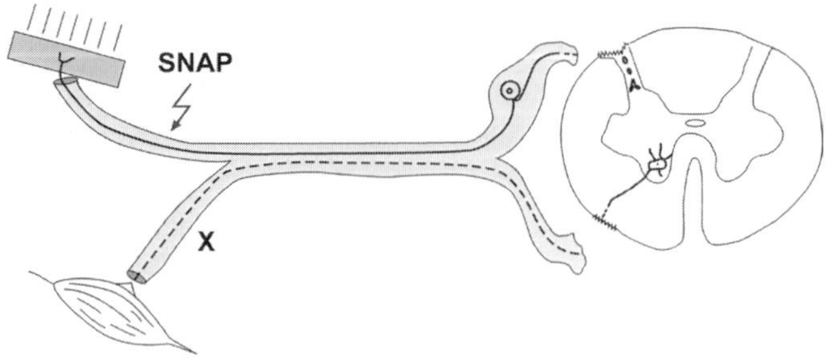

Fig. 7 Schematic drawing of root avulsions. SNAP can be elicited, as the sensory neuron with distal nerve fibre is intact.

the presence of sensory nerve action potentials (SNAPs) is the most reliable sign of a complete brachial plexus avulsion injury (Fig. 7).

Other ways of preoperatively diagnosing root avulsion by means of electrophysiology are to examine the muscles innervated by the dorsal primary branches of the pertinent spinal nerves (Bufalini and Pescatori 1969; Celli and Rovesta 1987). Reasonable correlations between this electrophysiological test and operative findings have been noted, but the overlap between adjacent myotomes causes difficulties in interpreting the outcome. Furthermore, as signs of muscle denervation in this context are quite late-appearing, the usefulness of this technique is very limited, particularly if intraspinal repair is considered.

Intraoperative electrophysiology. Evaluation of clinically nonfunctional spinal nerves is widely used, mainly as somatosensory evoked potentials (SEPs) (Landi *et al.* 1980). This allows us to test the usefulness of the proximal stump in a brachial plexus lesion as a site to base graft in reconstruction. It is also useful in cases where the plexus has not ruptured or is not pulled out of the intervertebral foramina, but is found in continuity. When there are no signs of distal function in terms of muscle response on electrical stimulation, it can be a most innocent neuropraxia lesion, which will recover spontaneously. Alternatively, it might be a most severe root avulsion injury, which occurred not as a pure traction injury but due to a central mechanism of shearing forces within the spinal canal (see Chap. 3).

If exploration is done early after the trauma, recordable SEPs indicate a favourable prognosis. However, there are limitations, as this test is sensitive to scarring and is not quantitative. Furthermore, this test assesses only the sensory or afferent connectivity into the central nervous system. As the ventral roots are more fragile than the dorsal roots (Bonney 1977; Privat *et al.* 1982), it is always possible that the SEPs gave a false-positive outcome, and futile attempts to restore motor function are performed (Fig. 9; Case 1 below). On the other hand, a false-negative SEP test, where the motor root is intact but the sensory root is avulsed (Fig. 9), although rarer and rather hypothetical, would make reconstructive surgery impossible.

Partial root avulsion affecting the ventral roots more than the dorsal roots has been reported to occur in about 10% of patients with avulsion injuries (Carvalho *et al.* 1997). To assess the status of the motor fibres in a root stump, it is possible to use the exclusive technique of motor evoked potentials (Turkof *et al.* 1997; Burkholder *et al.* 2003), which has not become routinely used. However, even when using these techniques, there are pitfalls such as the occurrence of afferent fibres in the ventral root (Hildebrand *et al.* 1997). Furthermore, electrophysiology does not allow for differentiation between incomplete avulsion and intact nerve roots, as a minor preserved part of the root is sufficient for conduction (Zhao *et al.* 1993). A negative response does not guarantee a lack of spinal nerve root anatomic continuity as assessed by intradural inspection (Oberle *et al.* 2002). If in doubt after such tests on a plexus found *in situ*, a conservative attitude is pertinent and a second intervention might prove necessary if there is no timely return of function.

Obviously, the status of the proximal stump, sometimes found deep in the intervertebral foramen, can be of dubious and uncertain quality, as long as an intraspinal exploration is not performed (Privat *et al.* 1982; Carvalho *et al.* 1997). However, a laminectomy should not be performed only to explore the intraspinal brachial plexus, but must always be performed with the intention to perform a root repair or reimplantation. Methods to further assess the situation of the proximal spinal nerve or root stumps in such difficult cases are, for instance, the histological assessment of myelinated fibres in the proximal stump (Malessy *et al.* 1999). Intraoperative electrophysiology together with histochemistry for the detection of the transmitter substance in motor neurons, choline acetyltransferase (CAT) (Hattori *et al.* 2004), is another way of further advancing the possibilities of a diagnosis of intraspinal lesions. Results can be difficult to interpret, however, as there might not always be a strict separation between afferent and efferent fibres in the roots (Hildebrand *et al.* 1997), and on account of the problem of interradicular connections (Schalow 1992). The logistics of coordinated activities between the operating theatre, the neurophysiologist, and the histopathologist can be quite cumbersome, difficult, and time-consuming; yet still leave the surgeon with an uncertainty regarding the diagnosis. In complement to the above efforts to gain an appreciation of the quality of a nerve stump, endoscopy procedures can be performed. An endoscope can be introduced through an adjacent empty foramen, which has been evacuated through the avulsion, to inspect the intraspinal connectivity of neighbouring roots (see Chap. 7, Fig. 1).

Spinal cord monitoring. It is of uttermost importance to monitor function in the spinal cord during manipulations for reimplantation (Owen 2004). The major purposes are to detect the onset of a surgically induced insult to the spinal cord, to provide information which can be used to modify the surgical technique, and to reverse the effect from an insult. In order to protect the ascending and descending fibre tracts, continuous assessments of the sensory and motor tracts are made. Although the somatosensory evoked potential (SEP) is commonly used, it does not reflect the situation in the ventral part of the spinal cord.

Reimplantation surgery is performed in the anterior part of the spinal cord, where the main spinal cord artery and motor tracts are particularly at risk. Transcranial motor evoked potential (MEP) is therefore used together with SEP. The MEP monitoring is 100% sensitive and specific; whereas the sensitivity of SEP monitoring has been reported to be unacceptably low, only 25%, and lagging behind the motor tract assessment (Hattori *et al.* 2004). Any change in the amplitude of monitoring should immediately prompt a response to prevent a surgically induced spinal cord injury by decompression, for instance, but also by raising the mean arterial pressure. An inadequate spinal cord perfusion caused by interference with the blood supply through compression or stretching is the most likely cause to spinal cord injury.

Imaging

Radiographs of the neck and upper thorax give valuable information regarding fractures and the possibility of cervical spine instability. Fractures of the transverse processes are associated with avulsion injury to the pertinent spinal nerve roots and traumatic insult to the vertebral artery (see below). Fracture dislocation of the first rib indicates a severe proximal or intraspinal lesion to the lower trunk of the plexus and to the subclavian artery. A raised hemidiaphragm on a chest X-ray reveals a most proximal C5 lesion.

Magnetic resonance imaging (MRI) is best used for visualisation of the extraspinal parts of the brachial plexus and for spinal cord lesions; whereas it is not optimal for considering individual roots (Hems *et al.* 1999), even after enhancement (Hayashi *et al.* 1998). A normal MRI of the supraclavicular plexus excludes significant postganglionic nerve disruption. In cases of plexus injury, the extradural findings of neuroma or fibrosis do not identify the exact site of injury, nor do they reliably distinguish between rupture and stretching (Hems *et al.* 1999). Direct evidence of root avulsion from the cord is limited by slice thickness. Ochi *et al.* (1994) used axial and axial oblique planes to predict root avulsion at the C5 and C6 levels. They achieved a diagnostic accuracy of 73% for C5 and 64% for C6, whereas Carvalho *et al.* (1997) found MRI to be unreliable in about 50% when compared to intradural inspection. Three-dimensional MR myelography (MRM) is a technique in which a myelogram-like image is produced by using a heavily T2-weighted sequence together with fat suppression. An accuracy rate of over 90% in detecting meningoceles and root avulsion was reported (Nakamura *et al.* 1997). Secondary MRI features associated with root avulsions are spinal cord oedema in the acute stage, lateral displacement of the spinal cord, posttraumatic syrinx, haemorrhage and scarring in the spinal canal, absence of roots in the canal or intervertebral foramina, and traumatic meningoceles. Indirect evidence of intraspinal plexus lesions can be obtained with this technique in the form of an increased signal on T2-weighted images of the denervated erector spinae muscles, at the earliest 2 weeks postinjury (Uetani *et al.* 1997). This technique, however, underestimates avulsions.

Myelography followed by computerised tomography (CT) appears to be the current imaging of choice for assessment of spinal nerve roots in centres where brachial plexus injuries are treated (Belzberg *et al.* 2004) (Fig. 8). A "negative" image of the roots on the

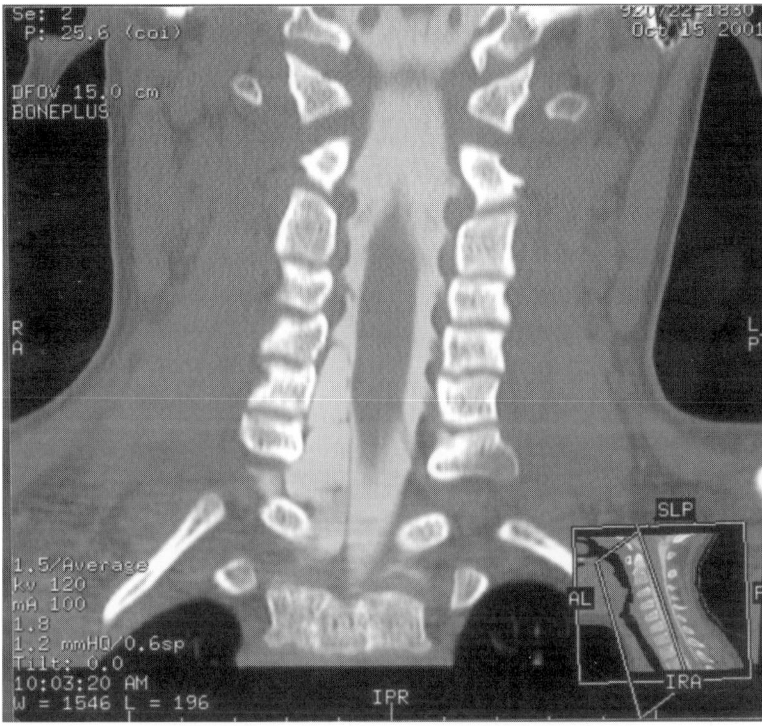

Fig. 8 CT myelogram of a complete C5–T1 brachial plexus avulsion lesion. Negative images of the roots are seen on the intact side, as well as cranial to the multiple meningoceles on the injured side.

normal side, appearing as lines in the opaque contrast (Marshall and De Silva 1986), should be visualised before the injured side can be assessed. Meningoceles occur only in about 60% of root avulsions (Fig. 8). When covering the spine from C3 to T2 by thin 2–3-mm slices, about 95% of the nerve roots can be displayed (Walker *et al.* 1996). The occurrence of partial avulsions of the ventral root with intact dorsal root (common), or avulsed dorsal root but intact ventral root (rare), can be seen with this technique (Fig. 9). However, it does not allow us to demonstrate the T1 roots and fully assess the C8 and T1 roots, due to beam hardening artefacts from the shoulders. As these lower roots run in a more oblique direction than the upper roots of the brachial plexus, they cannot be seen in continuity

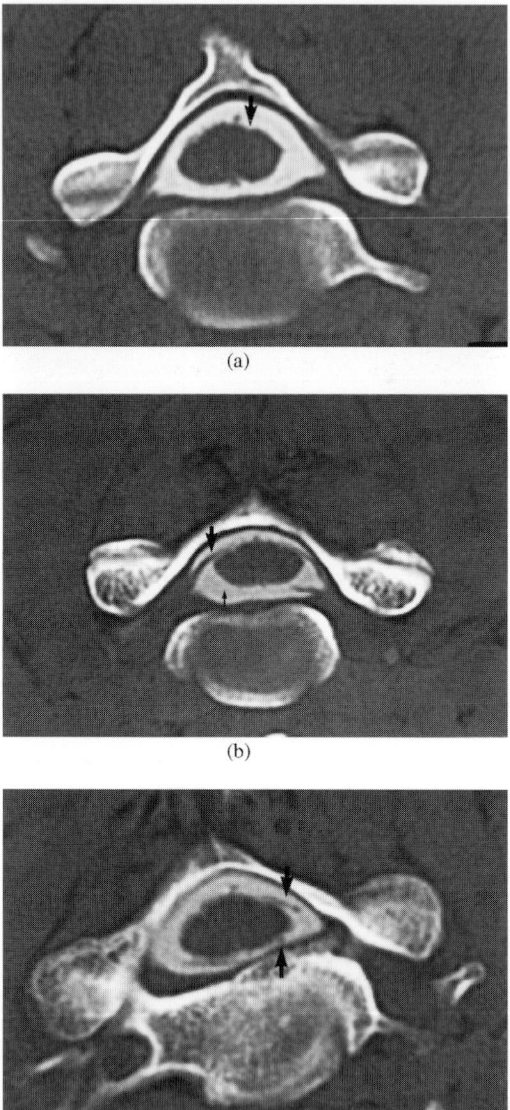

(a)

(b)

(c)

Fig. 9 CT myelograms. (a) Total avulsion with defect at the dorsal root–spinal cord junction (arrow). (b) Avulsion of the ventral root (small arrow) with intact dorsal root (large arrow). (c) Remaining dorsal root and stump of ventral root (arrows). (d) Avulsion of dorsal root with intact ventral root (arrow).

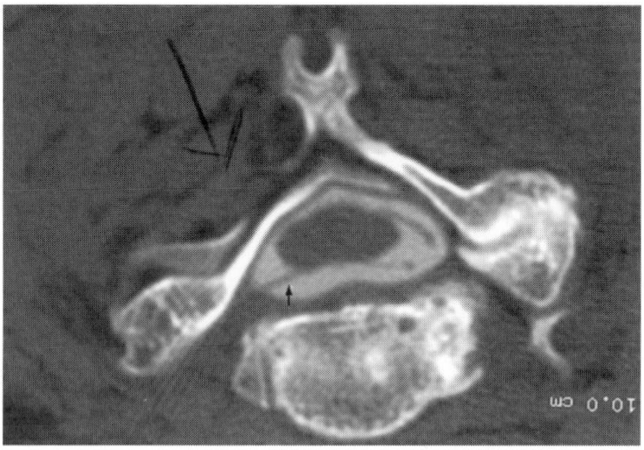

(d)

Fig. 9 (*Continued*)

from the cord to the foramen. This may result in false diagnosis or overdiagnosis of root avulsions.

The ideal outcome of such an assessment is a more than 95% specificity for root avulsion. The presence of a root stump on the surface of the spinal cord after a very proximal rupture, rather than avulsion, can sometimes be visualised if the CT myelogram is done early after the trauma (Hayashi *et al.* 1998; Hems *et al.* 1999; Tavakkolizadeh *et al.* 2001).

In lumbosacral plexus injuries, assessment by means of CT myelography is a much valued tool. Clinical diagnosis of the level of injury is difficult. Moreover, it is usually a severe trauma that has caused the nerve injury, which therefore is likely to be an intraspinal lesion. At the origin of the lumbosacral plexus, when the cauda equina ruptures rather than is avulsed from the conus (Chap. 3), there are possibilities to visualise proximal root stumps. This is done by mapping and tracing the roots on consecutive CT slides (Fig. 10).

CT myelography, being an invasive technique, can however be difficult to perform in the acute phase after a severe trauma. It can be most unpleasant for the patient, and potentially hazardous for those who have suffered a head trauma and have dura leakage from

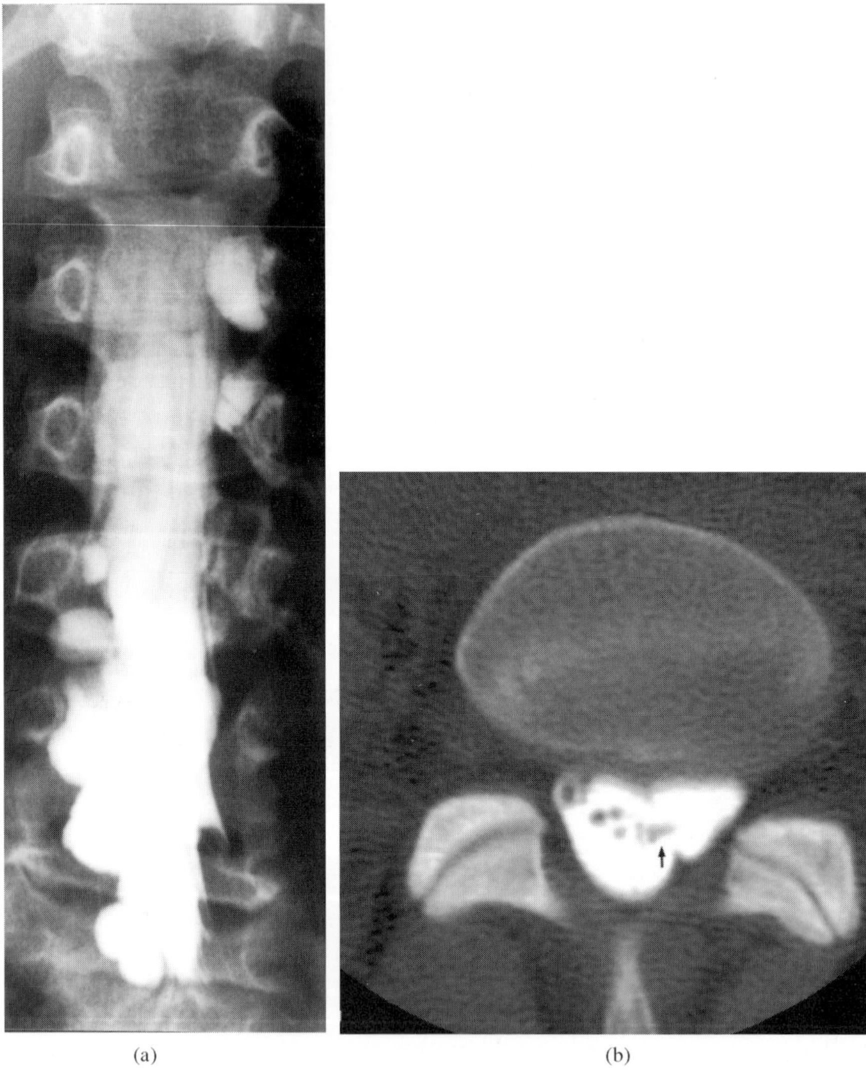

(a) (b)

Fig. 10 Myelogram and CT myelogram obtained of lumbosacral plexus lesions with meningoceles and ruptures of roots in the cauda equina. (a) Myelogram revealing numerous bilateral traumatic meningoceles with leakage of contrast material on the left from lumbar roots and on the right from L4 downward. (b) CT myelogram at the L5–S1 level revealing the few remaining roots and an anterior cyst in continuity with the subarachnoid space. Note the proximal root stump at the transition between the subarachnoid space and the cyst (arrow) available for reconstruction by means of nerve grafting (from Lang *et al*. 2004).

root avulsions. The outcome can be impossible to understand when there is severe contrast leakage and when the patient is dehydrated, which might be the case early after a trauma. Further development and refinement of MRI will, hopefully, replace myelography, which is often quite difficult for the patient.

Case 1. A 28-year-old man who sustained severe multi-trauma with bilateral arm and tibia fractures in a motorcycle accident had a clinically complete right-sided brachial plexus injury with a Horner sign, but no Tinel's sign. The CT myelography demonstrated clear avulsions with pseudomyelomeningoceles corresponding to C7, C8, and T1 spinal nerve roots. The dorsal roots of C5 and C6 could be seen, but not the corresponding ventral roots. Ventral root avulsions at those levels were suspected. The spinal cord appeared swollen, almost herniated, at the site of the surmised ventral root avulsion, indicating an effect of the trauma to the spinal cord (Fig. 11).

At surgery performed 6 days after the accident, the avulsion of C7–T1 could be confirmed, as the dorsal root ganglia and roots were found in the posterior triangle of the neck. There were 1–2 cm of good stumps at the foramina for C5 and C6. SEP gave a good response from those stumps, and they were consequently used for reconstruction in the hope that, in spite of the CT myelographic outcome, response could also be expected from the motor parts of those roots. However, shoulder and elbow function did not return. Obviously, a diagnosis of root avulsion is very difficult to make with certainty from an extraspinal exploration only. SEP does not reveal ventral root injury. There is a possibility of spinal cord injury to those spinal cord segments that have sustained root avulsion injury.

Case 2. Here is presented a case of vertebral artery thrombosis associated with brachial plexus injury, which indicates the preoperative use of magnetic resonance angiography (MRA). The vertebral artery is at risk from cervical spine trauma, which obviously is the case in severe brachial plexus injuries. A 27-year-old man sustained

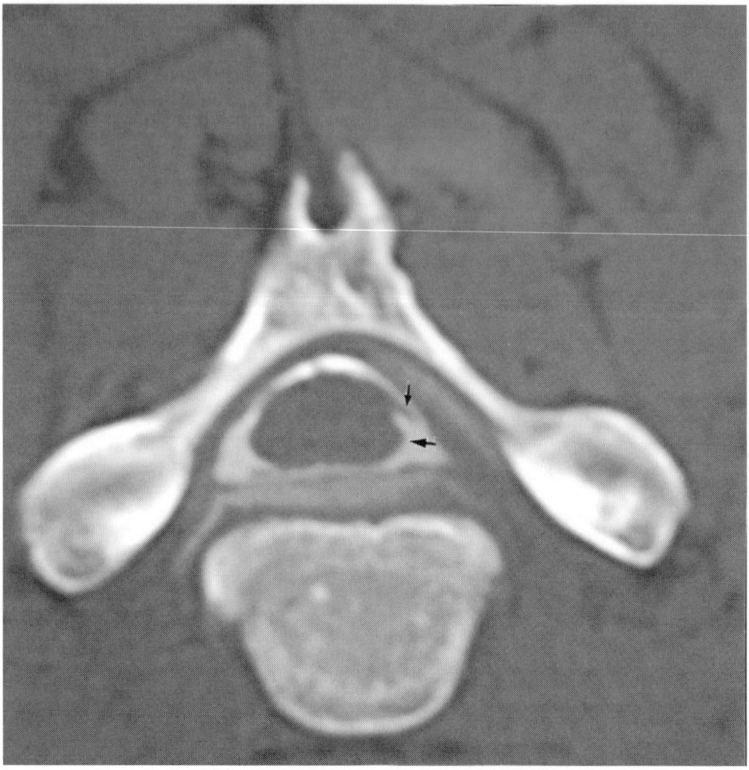

Fig. 11 Avulsion of ventral roots with cord swelling (large arrow). Intact dorsal root (small arrow).

a complete brachial plexus injury in a road traffic accident whilst on his motorcycle. He was subjected to trauma resuscitation, and trauma X-ray views of his cervical spine and chest were carried out. These demonstrated fractures ipsilateral to brachial plexus injury — fractures of the right transverse processes of C6, C7, and T1 — as well as fractures of the first and second ribs. He was referred 2 days after the accident for treatment of his right-sided brachial plexus injury. Preoperatively, he was found to be alert and orientated with a Glasgow coma score of 15. There was marked bruising in the posterior triangle of the neck. Examination of the cranial nerves was normal with the exception of a right Bernard–Horner syndrome. A right pan-plexus paralysis was noted with some residual power in the right trapezius and rhomboideus major. Altered sensation was present in the distribution of the fifth cervical dermatome with absent sensation in the dermatomes of C6, C7, C8, and T1. The Tinel's sign was absent.

CT myelography suggested complete avulsion of all five roots of the brachial plexus. The patient underwent surgery 2 days later. The procedure was lengthy. An incidental finding during surgery was visualisation of the vertebral artery, which appeared blue and thrombosed probably from intimal tear. During the course of the operation, it was noted that the patient had significant respiratory distress. Hence, postoperatively, intubation and ventilation were deemed necessary for 8 days. Further ventilatory support was required in the form of positive end expiratory pressure for a further 3 more days. Throughout the postoperative period, there were significant fluctuations in blood pressure and a pyrexia of 38 C. Blood cultures were negative.

When the patient was weaned off the ventilator, he was unable to move his right lower limb. Over the next 24 hours, a rapid recovery ensued. As the patient became ambulant, imbalance set in with the clinical signs of a rotatory nystagmus to the right and a positive Romberg's sign. Thrombocytosis with a platelet count of over 1000 was present.

A neurological opinion was sought to exclude an intracerebellar event, presumably secondary either to respiratory distress or from the presumed thrombosis of the vertebral artery. Magnetic resonance angiography (MRA) confirmed a complete occlusion of the right vertebral artery with good basilar circulation from the contralateral circulation (Fig. 12). As the platelet count was dropping and the patient was clinically improving, it was elected not to instigate antithrombotic therapy. The patient made a complete recovery and, when reviewed 6 weeks later, was noted — with the exception of the brachial plexus palsy and the Bernard–Horner sign — to be neurologically intact.

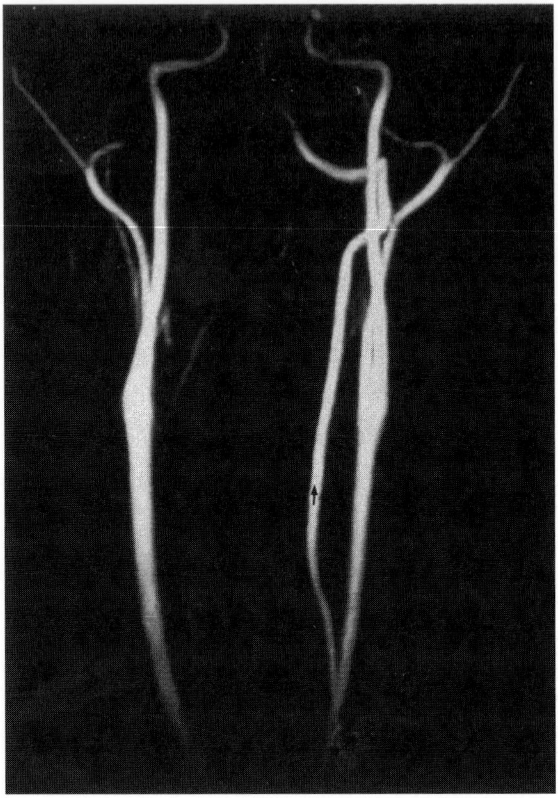

Fig. 12 MRA in a case of vertebral artery thrombosis after trauma to the neck with fractures of transverse processes and complete brachial plexus avulsion injury (the arrow indicates the vertebral artery on the unaffected side).

A preoperative protocol for patients intended for intraspinal brachial plexus surgery.

- Clinical assessment including history, as well as general and complete neurological examination (also of the lower extremities) for paralysis of peripheral and central type, i.e. Brown–Séquard syndrome.
- Full haematological and coagulation screening.
- Chest X-ray for the assessment of diaphragm paralysis.

- Cervical spine with flexion–extension views for occult instability and transverse process fractures.
- MRI of cervical spine for signs of spine instability, intraspinal haematoma, syrinx, and spinal cord injury.
- MRA to look for integrity of major proximal vessels, i.e. integrity of vertebral artery, and to exclude dissection aneurysm.
- CT myelogram for assessments of intraspinal or root injuries.

References

Belzberg AJ, Dorsi MJ, Storm PB, Moriarity JL, Surgical repair of brachial plexus injury: a multinational survey of experienced peripheral nerve surgeons, *J Neurosurg* **101**:365–376, 2004.

Bonney G, Some lesions of the brachial plexus, *Ann R Coll Surg Engl* **59**:298–306, 1977.

Bufalini C, Pescatori G, Posterior cervical electromyography in the diagnosis and prognosis of brachial plexus injuries, *J Bone Joint Surg* **51**:627–631, 1969.

Burkholder LM, Houlden DA, Midha R *et al.*, Neurogenic motor evoked potentials: role in brachial plexus surgery, *J Neurosurg* **98**:607–610, 2003.

Carvalho GA, Nikkhah G, Matthies C *et al.*, Diagnosis of root avulsions in traumatic brachial plexus injuries. The value of computerized tomography, myelography and magnetic resonance imaging, *J Neurosurg* **86**:69–76, 1997.

Celli L, Rovesta C, Electrophysiologic intraoperative evaluations of the damaged root in traction of the brachial plexus, in Terzis JK (ed.), *Microreconstruction of Nerve Injuries*, WB Saunders, Philadelphia, PA, pp. 437–482, 1987.

Frazier CH, Skillern PG, Supraclavicular subcutaneous lesion of the brachial plexus not associated with skeletal injuries, *JAMA* **57**:1957–1963, 1911.

Hattori Y, Doi K, Dhawan V *et al.*, Choline acetyltransferase activity and evoked spinal cord potentials for diagnosis of brachial plexus injury, *J Bone Joint Surg* **86**:70–73, 2004.

Hayashi N, Yamamato S, Okubo T *et al.*, Avulsion injury of cervical nerve roots: enhanced intradural nerve roots at MR imaging, *Radiology* **206**:817–822, 1998.

Hems T, Birch R, Carlstedt T, The role of magnetic resonance imaging in the management of traction injuries to the adult brachial plexus, *J Hand Surg* **24**:550–555, 1999.

Hildebrand C, Karlsson M, Risling M, Ganglionic axons in motor roots and pia mater, *Prog Neurobiol* **51**:89–128, 1997.

Landi A, Copeland SA, Parry CBW, Jones SJ, The role of somatosensory evoked potentials and nerve conduction studies in the surgical management of brachial plexus injuries, *J Bone Joint Surg* **62**:492–496, 1980.

Lang E, Borges J, Carlstedt T, Surgical treatment of lumbosacral plexus injuries, *J Neurosurg* **1**:64–71, 2004.

Malessy MJA, van Duinen SG, Feirabend HK *et al.*, Correlation between histopathological findings in C5 and C6 nerve stumps and motor recovery following nerve grafting for repair of brachial plexus injury, *J Neurosurg* **91**:636-644, 1999.

Marshall RW, De Silva RD, Computerised axial tomography in traction injuries of the brachial plexus, *J Bone Joint Surg* **68**:734–738, 1986.

Nakamura T, Yabe Y, Horiuchi Y *et al.*, Magnetic resonance myelography in brachial plexus injury, *J Bone Joint Surg* **79**:764–769, 1997.

Oberle J, Antoniadis G, Kast E, Richter HP, Evaluation of traumatic cervical nerve root injuries by intraoperative evoked potentials, *Neurosurgery* **51**:1182–1190, 2002.

Ochi M, Ikuta Y, Watanabe M *et al.*, The diagnostic value of MRI in traumatic brachial plexus injury, *J Hand Surg* **19**:55–59, 1994.

Owen JH, Intraoperative electrophysiologic monitoring of the spinal cord and nerve roots, in Winn HR (ed.), *Youman's Neurological Surgery*, 5th edn, Vol. 4, pp. 4203–4226, 2004.

Privat JM, Mailhe D, Allieu Y *et al.*, Précoce hémilaminectomie cervicale exploratrice et neurotisation du plexus brachial, in Simon L (ed.), *Plexus Brachial et Médecine de Rééducation*, Masson, Paris, France, pp. 66–73, 1982.

Robotti E, Longhi P, Verna G, Bocchiotti G, Brachial plexus surgery. An historical perspective, *Hand Clin* **11**:511–533, 1995.

Schalow G, Ventral root afferent and dorsal root efferent fibres in dog and human lower sacral nerve roots, *Gen Physiol Biophys* **11**:123–131, 1992.

Seddon HJ (ed.), *Peripheral Nerve Injuries*, Medical Research Council Special Report Series No. 282, Her Majesty's Stationery Office, London, 1954.

Tavakkolizadeh A, Saifuddin A, Birch R, Imaging of adult brachial plexus traction injuries, *J Hand Surg* **26**:183–191, 2001.

Turkof E, Millesi H, Turkof R *et al.*, Intraoperative electroneurodiagnostics (transcranial electrical motor evoked potentials) to evaluate the functional status of anterior spinal roots and spinal nerves during brachial plexus surgery, *Plast Reconstr Surg* **99**:1632–1641, 1997.

Uetani M, Hayashi K, Hashmi R *et al.*, Traction injury of the brachial plexus: signal intensity changes of the posterior cervical paraspinal muscles on MRI, *J Comput Assist Tomogr* **21**:790–795, 1997.

Walker AT, Chaloupka JC, de Lotbiniere ACJ *et al.*, Detection of nerve rootlet avulsion on CT myelography in patients with birth palsy and brachial plexus injury after trauma, *Am J Roentgenol* **167**:1283–1287, 1996.

Weddell G, Feinstein B, Pattle RE, The electrical activity of voluntary muscle in man under normal and pathological conditions, *Brain* **67**:178–252, 1944.

Zhao S, Kim DH, Kline DG *et al.*, Somatosensory evoked potentials induced by stimulating a variable number of nerve fibers in rat, *Muscle Nerve* **16**:1220–1227, 1993.

5

PALLIATIVE PERIPHERAL NERVE PROCEDURES FOR SPINAL ROOT INJURIES

The conventional approach to treat brachial plexus avulsion injuries has been to apply palliative, noncurative methods, i.e. transfers of nerves within or outside the brachial plexus to the avulsed roots or nerves in attempts to compensate for the loss of sensory and motor function. The possibility for palliative surgery decreases with the increase in number of root avulsions, i.e. with severity of the lesion. In cases of complete C5-to-T1 avulsions,which fortunately are quite rare (less than 10% of severe traumatic brachial plexus traction injuries), the possibility for palliative peripheral nerve surgery is also very limited. The current concept in this devastating type of spinal cord injury is to restore shoulder abduction by spinal accessory nerve to suprascapular nerve transfer and elbow flexion by intercostal nerve to musculocutaneous nerve transfer (Belzberg *et al.* 2004), although some surgeons would use the phrenic nerve and the contralateral C7 spinal nerve (Gu *et al.* 1989; Gu *et al.* 1992). Nerve transfers also have a place in combination with the intraspinal repair technique in order to optimise the chances of functional restoration in cases of complete avulsion injury (Carlstedt *et al.* 2004).

The principle of nerve transfers is old (cf. Narakas 1991). Harris and Low (1903) performed intraplexus transfers of ruptured spinal nerves and end-to-side repairs, which have now sparked renewed interest (Viterbo *et al.* 1992). Transfer of extraplexus nerves from the cervical plexus was first described by Tuttle (1912).

Intraplexus Transfers

Intraplexus transfers can be performed in cases of occasional root avulsions together with spinal nerve ruptures. One or two avulsed roots can be reconnected either directly or through nerve grafts to an adjacent ruptured spinal nerve. For instance, in cases of rupture of the C5 and C6 spinal nerves and avulsion of C7 with intact lower root to C8 and T1, the ventral root of C7 could be directly apposed to part of the trimmed cross-section area of the proximal stump of C6. Such intraplexus transfers could also be used with success when two spinal nerves are ruptured and two roots are avulsed, but should not be tried with fewer spinal nerve ruptures and more than two root avulsions.

The key functions of the arm, such as shoulder stability and elbow flexion, should have priority in regeneration (Narakas 1990; Kline and Hudson 1995). Too many diversions of regrowing axons directed at many various targets might lead to some reinnervation of many muscles, but with no functional gain. It is known, however, that there normally is some "reserve capacity" in the motor system that can, to a certain extent, be used and redirected by nerve transfers without any significant donor-site morbidity. A reduced number of motoneurons could maintain normal muscle power by enlargement of motor units (Gordon *et al.* 2003).

Extraplexus Transfers

Extraplexus transfers are possible from several nerves in the vicinity of the brachial plexus for irreparable lesions. The original use of nonplexus nerves in brachial plexus injuries was described by Seddon (1963), who successfully used intercostal nerves for elbow flexion. Transfers of the spinal, accessory, or XI nerve and of the fascicles of the ulnar nerve to the branch of the musculocutaneous nerve for biceps are, together with the intercostal nerves, the most common nerve transfers. Fascicles of the fully functional ulnar nerve are, in cases of avulsion injuries to the upper part of the brachial plexus with intact lower roots, transferred to the motor branch of the biceps muscle in order to gain elbow flexion (Oberlin *et al.* 1994). This is a procedure not really applicable in cases of more extensive avulsion injuries, which are considered for intraspinal repair; but is quite useful in adult cases of upper brachial plexus avulsion injuries, i.e. C5–C6 (although it is disappointing when the C7 nerve has also been avulsed). This transfer has proved disappointing in obstetrical cases.

Intercostal Nerve Transfers

Intercostal nerve transfers use the upper nerves T3–T6, which are approached through an incision from the upper arm, across the axilla, and along the chest wall behind the pectoralis major to the level of the nipple. The distal part of the infraclavicular brachial plexus in the axilla is exposed. The neurovascular bundle for the serratus anterior muscle is defined along the chest wall. The plane of the serratus anterior and its anterior parts is followed up to where the cutaneous branches of the intercostal nerves are found. These are traced proximally and deep into the muscle and to the inferior border of the rib. The origin of the external intercostal muscles is detached from the rib and the deep branch of the intercostal nerves found, sometimes after some "fishing" with a nerve hook. The nerve is then followed in anterior and posterior directions, usually with some irritating bleeding from the accompanying vessels. It is of course necessary to make sure, by means of a chest X-ray, that the pleura has not been breached during the dissection. In patients who have sustained rib fractures, this dissection could be difficult, if not impossible. If there is a phrenic nerve palsy only, the sensory branches of the intercostal or intercostobrachial nerves should be used. Sufficient length of the nerve should be mobilised in order to reach without tension to the intended recipient nerve, in most cases the musculocutaneous nerve (Malessy *et al.* 1993). A good transfer using intercostal nerves is to the long thoracic nerve for shoulder blade stability. This is an easy transfer that, in most cases, yields a good outcome, necessary for other palliative procedures at the shoulder (for instance, arthrodesis).

The intercostal nerve transfer is not only used for restoration of muscle function, but has also found a particular application in the alleviation of the severe pain that follows root avulsion injuries (Berman *et al.* 1998). In such cases, the intercostal nerves are joined to the cut surface of the ulnar or, more rarely, the median nerve. For the same purpose, supraclavicular nerves can be transferred to the sensory part of avulsed C7, C8, or T1 spinal nerves (Fig. 1). This is best done by dissecting the sensory or dorsal root from the ventral root. The dorsal root ganglion must be removed in order to clear the peripheral sensory conduit from its original and still intact axons, and allow for regrowth of centrally connected sensory nerve fibres from the transferred nerves.

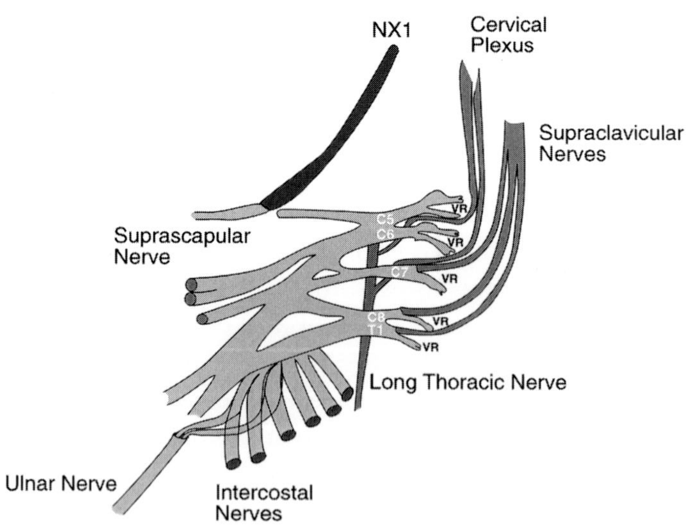

Fig. 1 Nerve transfers used in conjunction with intraspinal repair of complete C5–T1 brachial plexus avulsions. NXI (accessory) nerve to suprascapular nerve; cervical plexus to long thoracic nerve; supraclavicular nerves to sensory parts of lower cervical spinal nerves; and intercostal nerves to ulnar nerve.

Spinal Accessory Nerve Transfers

Transfer of the spinal accessory (NXI) nerve to the suprascapular or musculocutaneous nerves, preserving the upper branches to the trapezius, was described by Kotani *et al.* (1972) and Allieu (1989). For neurotisation, the most distal part of the accessory to be reached on the anterior aspect of the trapezius muscle, where branches of the transverse cervical artery enter into the muscle, is the site where the nerve is divided. It is mobilised in order to reach to a direct apposition to the suprascapular nerve, which has been dissected from the upper trunk of the brachial plexus (Fig. 1).

The accessory nerve is regularly used as part of the surgical strategy for total brachial plexus avulsion injury, together with spinal cord reimplantation. The transverse skin incision in the posterior triangle of the neck extended to the dorsal aspect of the midcervical spine for exploration of the extraspinal and intraspinal brachial plexus crosses the trajectory of the accessory spinal nerve. It is exposed after the skin and subcutaneous flaps have been raised at the upper anterior border of the trapezius muscleor even more proximally, as it leaves the sternocleidomastoid muscle. It is important to define this nerve before the approach to the lateral mass of the spine, as this approach should be posterior to the accessory nerve, but through the most anterior part of the trapezius muscle (see Chap. 7).

Other Nerves

Other nerves usable for transfers in cases of complete brachial plexus avulsion injury are the nerves from the cervical plexus (Brunelli 1980; Rutowski 1993), the phrenic nerve (Gu *et al.* 1989), the hypoglossal nerve (Slooff and Blauuw 1995), and the contralateral C7 spinal nerve (Gu *et al.* 1992).

The cervical plexus transfer offers some additional power to denervated muscles after complete brachial plexus avulsion injury (Carlstedt *et al.* 2004), but the branches of this plexus are quite minute, with a limited number of nerve fibres. The phrenic nerve, the hypoglossal nerve, and the contralateral C7 have not been used in conjunction with intraspinal repair. The hypoglossal nerve is not good for neurotisation of the brachial plexus, and there is some very severe donor-site morbidity from this procedure (Malessy *et al.* 1999). The functional outcome of contralateral C7 transfer is dubious with a limited motor recovery, a difficult relearning period to gain independent use of the recovery from activity on the donor site, and the risk of considerable donor-site morbidity (Ali *et al.* 2002; Midha 2004). Animal models for studies of neuropathic pain usually employ the cutting of a single spinal nerve. The risk of neuropathic pain following the use of contralateral C7 for nerve transfer procedures is therefore highly relevant (Ali *et al.* 2002). There is a pulmonary price to be paid when using the phrenic nerve (Chuang *et al.* 1995).This is obvious in patients who have sustained an injury to this nerve, and this transfer should not be used at all in obstetrical brachial plexus injuries.

Outcome of Nerve Transfers

The outcome of nerve transfers in brachial plexus surgery depends on several conditions (Merrell *et al.* 2001):

(1) Transfer from one motor nerve to another motor nerve, to limit sensory and motor mismatching during regeneration.
(2) Transfer without intervening nerve graft.
(3) Transfer for synergistic function, e.g. shoulder elevation and shoulder abduction (accessory to suprascapular nerve transfer).
(4) Transfer to nerve close to target muscle. This is favourable when transferring the fascicles of the ulnar nerve to the muscle branch of the musculocutaneous nerve; but less so in transfer from intercostal to biceps nerve, or from accessory to suprascapular nerve, as the most distal part of the donor nerve must be used in order to reach to the recipient nerve without a nerve graft.

In some instances, this peripheral nerve surgery results in a function return as good as with nerve grafting repair of ruptured spinal nerves in the brachial plexus (Htut *et al.* 2007). However, the use of nerve transfers as a remedy in plexus lesions is not always successful. Transfer from the intercostal nerve to the biceps nerve succeeds in restoring biceps function in about only 60% of cases (Merrell *et al.* 2001). The accessory nerve is useful only for transfer to the suprascapular nerve, as any other target nerve (e.g. the axillary or musculocutaneous nerve) would require a nerve graft with documented functional limitations (Chuang *et al.* 1995; Merrell *et al.* 2001). In the use for shoulder function, transfer from the accessory to the suprascapular nerve can be expected to result in shoulder stability and limited abduction (Narakas 1995; Chuang *et al.* 1995; Birch *et al.* 1998); but external rotation, the important shoulder function used to steer the arm (Alnot *et al.* 1998), is seldom or never restored (Narakas 1991; Bentolila *et al.* 1999; Oberlin 2000). There is a small possibility that both the supraspinatus and infraspinatus muscle functions can be restored from accessory or any other nerve transfer. This deficit in palliative nerve surgery has been suggested to depend on a lack of synergism or plasticity in order to allow for a "re-education" leading to a new voluntary control (Malessy *et al.* 2003).

There is obviously very little, if any at all, plasticity within the spinal cord for a change in motor control (Carlstedt *et al.* 2004), but there is a requirement for cerebral plasticity to make the transfer functionally effective (Malessy *et al.* 1998; Malessy *et al.* 2003). The possibility of success is therefore greater when there are already central but "silent" parallel circuits, which become active after a peripheral nerve surgery. This happens, for instance, after intercostal to biceps transfer, but is less efficient when such preformed "reserve" central connections do not exist or when the transfer is asked to perform multiple or complicated tasks. Even when the conditions are favourable regarding cortical plasticity and simple new movements, such as when trying to perform elbow flexion after an intercostal nerve transfer, there is never going to be full or normal activity, as respiration will permanently influence movements. Moreover, there is always a certain degree of donor-site morbidity. For some transfers, this does not disturb a useful function and can be a reasonable price to pay, if there is a functional gain within the denervated extremity, i.e. a muscle power of M3 or more. But, in other types of transfers, the function loss is too severe and the regeneration of activity will please only the surgeon.

In complete brachial plexus avulsion injuries, the option of nerve transfers is limited because the number of nerves to repair is always higher than the available donor nerves. There are simply not enough resources for nerve transfers. There is little recovery in the proximal part of the arm from nerve transfers in such cases, and hand function cannot be restored by this technique. This is in contrast to the encouraging outcome from spinal cord reimplantation of avulsed roots where hand function can be achieved (Carlstedt *et al.* 2004; see Chap. 8). However, nerve transfers can be useful in combination with repair strategies of the avulsed nerve roots.

End-to-Side or Termino-Lateral Repair

End-to-side or termino-lateral repair has been advocated to augment the number of available nerve fibres for restoration of function (Viterbo *et al.* 1992; Lundborg *et al.* 1994). This technique is based on the hypothesis that intact nerve fibres in an intact donor nerve would, after being offered a new and alternative conduit, send out new fibres by sprouting sideways into the attached nerve graft maintaining their original innervation. However, there is little to support such a hypothesis. The internal environment in an uninjured peripheral nerve might be as nonpermissive to new axonal growth as is the central nervous system. There are growth inhibitory substances like condroitin sulphate proteoglycans (CSPGs) and myelin-associated glycoprotein (MAG) within the normal nerve that inhibit axonal sprouting (Mirsky and Jessen 1999; Zuo *et al.* 1998). Not until the nerve has been injured, inducing a change in Schwann cell phenotype with the upregulation of regeneration-associated genes, are the conditions favourable for new axonal growth within the nerve.

A "perineural window" seems necessary for the achievement of such regeneration. This obviously would compromise the internal milieu of the nerve, which is essential for a preserved normal function (Spencer *et al.* 1975). Breaching the perineurium is likely to injure nerve fibres in the donor nerve, with the consequence of an end-to-end type of regeneration rather than an end-to-side growth. Muscle reinnervation by a new and extra axon branch from a nerve fibre still in contact with its original target would most likely induce unwanted and counterproductive cocontractions between the original and the newly innervated muscles. This technique has therefore come into disrepute as a clinically useful strategy (Rowan *et al.* 2000).

A more extreme approach to functional deficits after complete brachial plexus avulsion injuries is the double free-muscle transfer technique (Doi *et al.* 1995). This technique does not increase the possibility of more function, as it depends on what nerves are available for reconstruction, but it is of course an option in long-standing desolate cases (Barrie *et al.* 2004).

Lumbosacral Plexus Lesions

Lumbosacral plexus lesions are as devastating for function in the hip and leg as a severe brachial plexus injury is for function in the upper extremity. The most basic requirements for standing and walking are hip and knee stability and flexion. These key functions depend on sufficient power in proximal muscles such as the iliopsoas, the quadriceps, and the glutei muscles. Unlike the upper extremity, in which hand function is crucial, it would still be possible to stand and walk with impaired intrinsic muscle function or even loss of sensation in the foot. Therefore, in the case of complete and severe lumbosacral plexus injury, if function in a few proximal leg and hip muscles is recovered, the situation for the patient may dramatically change from being in a wheelchair to being able to stand and walk independently.

In cases where intraspinal repair of lumbosacral plexus lesion is impossible, e.g. when there is no proximal ventral root stump to use for reconstruction, it is possible to perform nerve transfers. The lower intercostal nerves can be rerouted to the femoral nerve in cases of severe lumbar plexus injury. This has been studied experimentally in rats (Zhao *et al.* 1997), and has been found to give a functional effect.

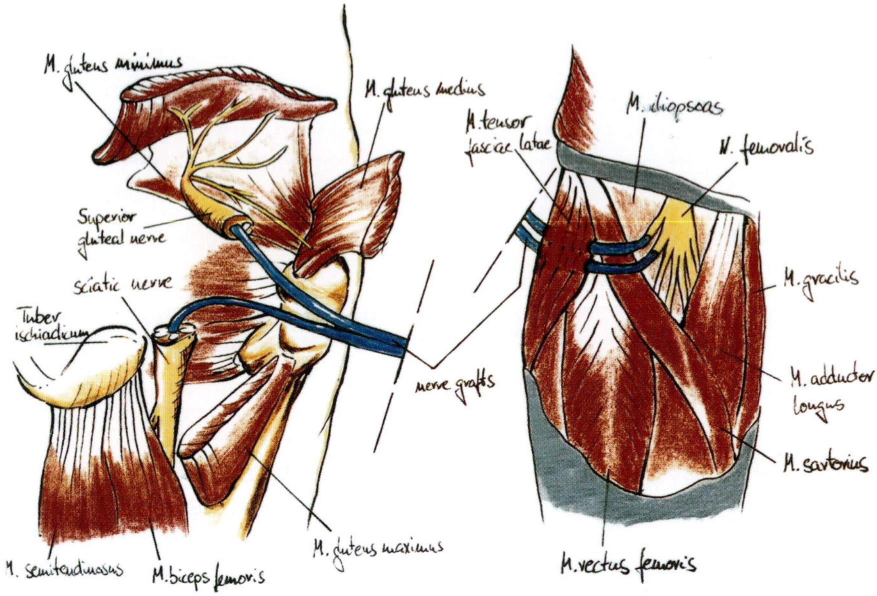

Fig. 2 Transfer of fascicles from intact femoral nerve to gluteal and sciatic nerves in cases of irreparable sacral plexus lesions (from Lang *et al.* 2004).

It has also been applied in humans with severe intraspinal lumbar plexus injury and proved to be efficient (Lang *et al.* 2004). A palliative method using branches of the glutei muscles for hip stability has been developed. Two to three fascicles from the intact ipsilateral femoral nerve can, through nerve grafts, reach and connect to the inferior gluteal nerve or the sciatic nerve with functional gain (Fig. 2).

An illustrative case

An illustrative case of severe lumbosacral plexus injury, which was treated with palliative peripheral nerve transfers, is that of a 5-year-old girl with bilateral injuries sustained in a road traffic accident. The girl was hit by a car and sustained serious injuries to the lower part of her abdomen and pelvis fractures with a sacral plexus lesion on the right side and a lumbar plexus lesion on the left side. Clinically, there was no activity in the quadriceps and adductor muscles on the left side. On the right side, there was mainly loss of activity of the

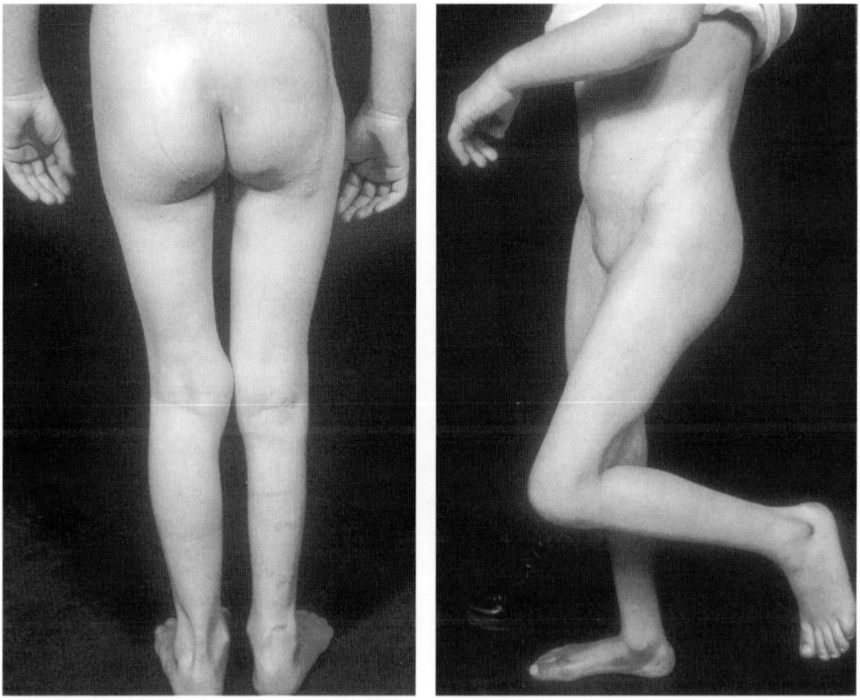

(a) (b)

Fig. 3 A case of severe bilateral lumbosacral plexus lesions: outcome from intercostal to lumbar plexus nerve transfer (left leg) and fascicles from intact femoral nerve to gluteal nerves (right leg). (a) There is ability to stabilise hips and knees to stand independently. (b) Stability in recovered muscles in the right hip supports one leg standing, and activity in iliopsoas muscle allows for hip flexion. Note scars from transfers (from Lang *et al.* 2004).

sacral plexus. On this side, there was normal activity in the femoral nerve, but weak activity in the obturator nerve. There was no hip stability and no hamstring or muscle function distal to the knee on the right side. There was also loss of hip flexion and knee extension on the left side. The patient was unable to stand and walk without support. A CT myelogram demonstrated an avulsion or intraspinal injury of the nerve roots of the sacral plexus on the right side and a lumbar plexus lesion on the left side (Chap. 4, Fig. 10).

At surgery, the sciatic and superior gluteal nerves of the right side were identified, but showed no response to stimulation. The lateral part of the femoral nerve supplying the lateral portions of the quadriceps muscle was separated from the main trunk of the femoral nerve, as distal as possible. These two nerve fascicles were cut to receive nerve grafts. The sural nerve grafts were positioned in the region of the femoral nerve and then tunnelled underneath the tensor fasciae latae muscle into the wound on the back of the hip. Of the two strands of the nerve graft that were reconnected to the two femoral fascicles, one was applied to the superior gluteal nerve and the other to the medial part of the sciatic nerve (Fig. 2).

The lesioned lumbar plexus of the left side was reinnervated with nerve grafts from the lower intercostal nerves. The femoral nerve was dissected proximally onto the lumbar spine. The intercostal nerves 10 and 11 were dissected free and cut proximally in order to obtain as many motor nerve fibres as possible. They were reconnected intra-abdominally to the proximal part of the femoral nerve.

There was recovery in muscle function in both legs, which resulted in the patient's ability to stand and walk independently after 1.5 years (cf. Lang *et al.* 2004) (Fig. 3).

Conclusion

The palliative procedures used together with intraspinal repair in cases of complete brachial plexus avulsion injury C5–T1 are transfers of the accessory nerve to the suprascapular nerve for shoulder joint stability and limited abduction; transfers of one or more branches from the cervical plexus (or of a couple of intercostal nerves) to the long thoracic nerve for shoulder blade stability; transfers of supraclavicular sensory nerves to the postganglionic part of the dorsal root of C7, C8, or T1 (Carlstedt *et al.* 2004); and intercostal nerve transfers to the ulnar nerve. The last two transfers are mainly for the prevention or alleviation of severe avulsion pain (Fig. 1).

In cases of severe intraspinal or extraspinal lumbar plexus injuries, where a direct repair is impossible due to nonexisting or unapproachable proximal stumps, lower intercostal nerves are transferred to the femoral nerve for knee extension and stability. In cases of complete and nonreparable sacral plexus lesions, fascicles from the femoral nerve are transferred to the superior gluteal nerve for hip stability (Fig. 2).

References

Ali Z, Meyer RA, Belzberg AJ, Neuropathic pain after C7 spinal nerve transection in man, *Pain* **96**:41–47, 2002.

Allieu Y, Les neurotisations par le nerf spinal dans les avulsions du plexus brachial de l'adulte, in Alnot JY, Narakas AO (eds.), *Les Paralysies du Plexus Brachial*, Monographie du Groupe de l'Etude de la Main, Expansion Scientifique Française, Paris, France, pp. 173–179, 1989.

Alnot JY, Rostoucher P, Oberlin C, Touam C, Les paralysies traumatiques C5–C6 et C5–C6–C7 du plexus brachial de l'adulte par lésions supraclaviculaires, *Rev Chir Orthop Reparatrice Appar Mot* **84**:113–123, 1998.

Barrie KA, Steinman SP, Shrin AY *et al.*, Gracilis free muscle transfer for restoration of function after complete brachial plexus avulsion, *Neurosurg Focus* **16**:article 8, 2004.

Belzberg AJ, Dorsi MJ, Storm PB, Moriarity JL, Surgical repair of brachial plexus injury: a multinational survey of experienced peripheral nerve surgeons, *J Neurosurg* **101**:365–376, 2004.

Bentolila V, Nizard R, Bizot P, Sedel L, Complete traumatic brachial plexus palsy, *J Bone Joint Surg [Am]* **81**:27–28, 1999.

Berman JS, Birch R, Anand P, Pain following human brachial plexus injury with spinal cord root avulsion and the effect of surgery, *Pain* **75**:199–207, 1998.

Birch R, Bonney G, Wynn Parry CBW, *Surgical Disorders of the Peripheral Nerves*, Churchill Livingstone, London, p. 539, 1998.

Brunelli G, Neurotization of avulsed roots of the brachial plexus by means of anterior nerves of the cervical plexus, *Int J Microsurg* **2**:55–58, 1980.

Carlstedt T, Anand P, Htut M *et al.*, Restoration of hand function and so called "breathing arm" after intraspinal repair of C5–T1 brachial plexus avulsion injury, *Neurosurg Focus* **16**:article 7, 2004.

Chuang D, Lee G, Hashen F *et al.*, Restoration of shoulder abduction by nerve transfer in avulsion brachial plexus injury: evaluation of 99 patients with various nerve transfers, *Plast Reconstr Surg* **96**:122–128, 1995.

Doi K, Sakai X, Kuwata K *et al.*, Double free muscle transfer to restore prehension following complete brachial plexus avulsion, *J Hand Surg [Am]* **20**:408–414, 1995.

Gordon T, Sulaiman O, Boyd G, Experimental strategies to promote functional recovery after peripheral nerve injuries, *J Peripher Nerv Syst* **8**:236–250, 2003.

Gu YD, Wu MM, Zhen YL *et al.*, Phrenic nerve transfer for brachial plexus motor neurotisation, *Microsurgery* **10**:287–289, 1989.

Gu YD, Zhang GM, Chen DS *et al.*, Seventh cervical nerve root transfer from the contralateral healthy side for treatment of brachial plexus root avulsion, *J Hand Surg* **17**:518–521, 1992.

Harris W, Low VW, On the importance of accurate muscular analysis in lesions of the brachial plexus and treatment of Erb's palsy and infantile paralysis of the upper extremity by cross-union of nerve roots, *Br Med J* **2**:1035–1038, 1903.

Htut M, Misra VP, Anand P *et al.*, Motor recovery and the breathing arm after brachial plexus surgical repairs, including re-implantation of avulsed spinal roots into the spinal cord, *J Hand Surg [Br]* **32**:170–178, 2007.

Kline DG, Hudson AR, *Nerve Injuries: Operative Results for Major Nerve Injuries, Entrapments, and Tumors*, WB Saunders, Philadelphia, PA, p. 611, 1995.

Kotani PT, Matsuda H, Suzuki T, Trial surgical procedures of nerve transfers to avulsion injuries of the brachial plexus, *Excerpta Med* **291**:348–351, 1973. Proceedings of the 12th Congress of SICOT, Tel Aviv, Israel, October 9–12, 1972.

Lang E, Borges J, Carlstedt T, Surgical treatment of lumbosacral plexus injuries, *J Neurosurg* **1**:64–71, 2004.

Lundborg G, Zhao Q, Kanje M *et al.*, Can sensory and motor collateral sprouting be induced from intact peripheral nerve by end-to-side anastomosis?, *J Hand Surg* **19**:277–282, 1994.

Malessy MJA, Bakker D, Dekker AJ *et al.*, Functional magnetic resonance imaging and control over the biceps muscle after intercostal–musculocutaneous nerve transfer, *J Neurosurg* **98**:261–268, 2003.

Malessy MJA, van der Kamp W, Thomeer RTWM *et al.*, Cortical excitability of the biceps muscle after intercostal-to-musculocutaneous nerve transfer, *Neurosurgery* **42**:787–795, 1998.

Malessy MJA, van Dijk JG, Thomeer RWTM, Respiration-related activity in the biceps brachii muscle after intercostal–musculocutaneous nerve transfer, *Clin Neurol Neurosurg* **95**(Suppl):95–102, 1993.

Malessy MJA, van Duinen SG, Feirabend HK *et al.*, Correlation between histopathological findings in C5 and C6 nerve stumps and motor recovery following nerve grafting for repair of brachial plexus injury, *J Neurosurg* **91**:636-644, 1999.

Merrell GA, Barrie KA, Katz DL *et al.*, Results of nerve transfer for restoration of shoulder and elbow function in the context of meta-analysis of the English literature, *J Hand Surg* **26**:303–314, 2001.

Midha R, Nerve transfers for severe brachial plexus injuries: a review, *Neurosurg Focus* **16**:article 5, 2004.

Mirsky R, Jessen KR, The neurobiology of Schwann cells, *Brain Pathol* **9**:293–311,1999.

Narakas AO, Brachial plexus injuries, in McCarthy JG, May JW, Littler WJ (eds.), *Plastic Surgery*, Vol. 3, Saunders, Philadelphia, PA, pp. 4776–4816, 1990.

Narakas AO, Compression and traction neuropathies about the shoulder and arm, in Gelberman RH (ed.), *Operative Nerve Repair and Reconstruction*, JB Lippincott, Philadelphia, PA, pp. 1147–1176, 1991.

Narakas AO, Examen du patient et de la fonction des divers groupes musculaires du membre supérieur, in Alnot JY, Narakas AO (eds.), *Les Paralysies du Plexus Brachial*, 2nd edn, Expansion Scientifique Française, Paris, France, pp. 52–67, 1995.

Oberlin C, *Manuel de Chirurgie du Membre Supérieur*, Elsevier, Paris, France, pp. 193–198, 2000.

Oberlin C, Beal D, Leechavengvongs S *et al.*, Nerve transfer to biceps muscle using a part of ulnar nerve for C5–C6 avulsion of the brachial plexus. Anatomical study and report of four cases, *J Hand Surg* **19**:232–237, 1994.

Rowan PR, Chen LE, Urbinak JR, End-to-side nerve repair. A review, *Hand Clin* **16**:151–159, 2000.

Rutowski R, Neurotizations by means of the cervical plexus in over 100 patients with from one to five root avulsions of the brachial plexus, *Microsurgery* **14**:285–288, 1993.

Seddon HJ, Nerve grafting, *J Bone Joint Surg* **45**:447–461, 1963.

Slooff ACJ, Blauuw G, Aspects particuliers, in Alnot JY, Narakas AO (eds), *Les Paralysies du Plexus Brachial*, 2nd edn, Monographie de la Société Française de Chirurgie de la main, Expansion Scientifique Française, Paris, France, pp. 282–284, 1995.

Spencer PS, Weinberg HJ, Raine CS, Prineas JW, The perineurial window — a new model of focal demyelination and remyelination, *Brain Res* **96**:323–329, 1975.

Tuttle H, Exposure of the brachial plexus with nerve transplantation, *J Am Med Assoc* **61**:15–17, 1912.

Viterbo F, Trindade JC, Hoshino K *et al.*, Latero-terminal neurorrhaphy without removal of the epineural sheath. Experimental study in rats, *Rev Paul Med* **110**:267–275, 1992.

Zhao S, Beuerman RW, Kline DG, Neurotization of motor nerves innervating the lower extremity by utilizing the lower intercostal nerves, *J Reconstr Microsurg* **113**:39–45, 1997.

Zuo J, Hernandez YJ, Muir D, Chondroitin sulphate proteoglycan with neurite-inhibiting activity is up-regulated following peripheral nerve injury, *J Neurobiol* **34**:41–54, 1998.

6

BASIC SCIENCE OF EXPERIMENTAL ROOT INJURIES

The Transitional Region (TR)

The interface between the peripheral nervous system (PNS) and the central nervous system (CNS), the transitional region (TR), is of conceptual importance in spinal nerve root avulsion injury. This is the usual site of rupture from a root traction trauma (Livesey and Fraher 1992). In the TR, axonal growth-promoting PNS tissue intermingles with growth-inhibitory CNS tissue. After injury, nerve cells cannot negotiate an elongation across the TR (Fig. 1) and grow into or out of the spinal cord (Oorschot and Jones 1990; Carlstedt 1997), as the TR is most effective in preventing regeneration. Knowing the normal structure and understanding reactions to root injury in the TR are therefore of importance for the surgical treatment and outcome of spinal root injuries.

The TR is characterised by the presence of a projection of CNS tissue from the spinal cord together with PNS tissue in the most proximal part of the root (Fig. 2). The contour of the CNS projection is usually dome- or cone-shaped with a peripherally oriented convexity (Berthold and Carlstedt 1977). In cervical ventral roots, the PNS–CNS interface is situated beneath the surface of the spinal cord (Fraher 1978; Fraher 1992). The CNS part of the root is dominated by fibrous astrocyte cell bodies and a dense network of astrocyte processes. The occurrence of astrocytes is about 10 times as high as that

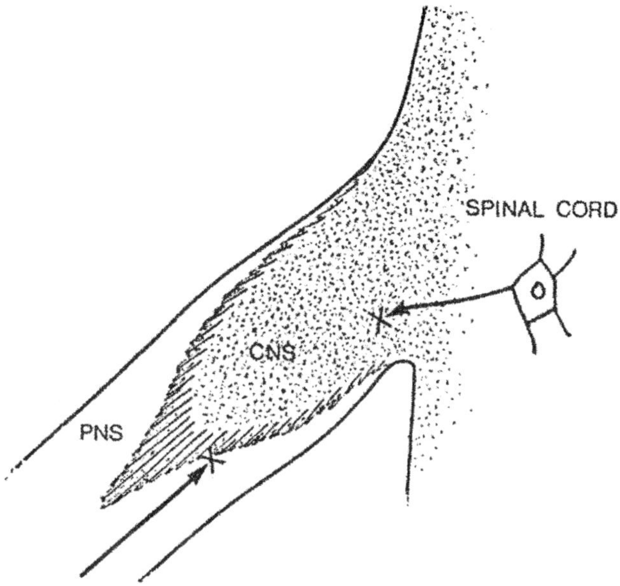

Fig. 1 Growth of lesioned nerve fibres and axons from intrinsic spinal cord neurons is impeded at the PNS–CNS interface in the dorsal root of the adult animal (from Carlstedt *et al.* 1989).

of the white matter or the glia limitans at the surface of the spinal cord. The CNS part of the root forms a fringe of astrocytic processes that projects about 100 μm distally among the nerve fibres (Fig. 2). Closer to the CNS part of the root, the astrocytic fringe becomes thicker, separating or enclosing individual myelinated nerve fibres in a tube- or holster-like fashion. In this way, a large myelinated fibre is situated in a "cul-de-sac" of PNS endoneurial space at the CNS part of the root (Fig. 3). This fringe acts as multiple channels or scaffolds for the nerve fibres at the PNS–CNS transition.

There is a particularly extensive reorganisation of dorsal root nerve fibres as they approach the CNS part of the root. This part of the root seems to act as a sieve, organising fibres according to size, and thereby function, in preparation for their entrance into different fibre tracts of the spinal cord. The largest fibres become directed to the centre of the root, whereas the thinly myelinated and unmyelinated fibres are relocated to the periphery of the root and concentrated to the ventrolateral zone of each rootlet (Fig. 4). This

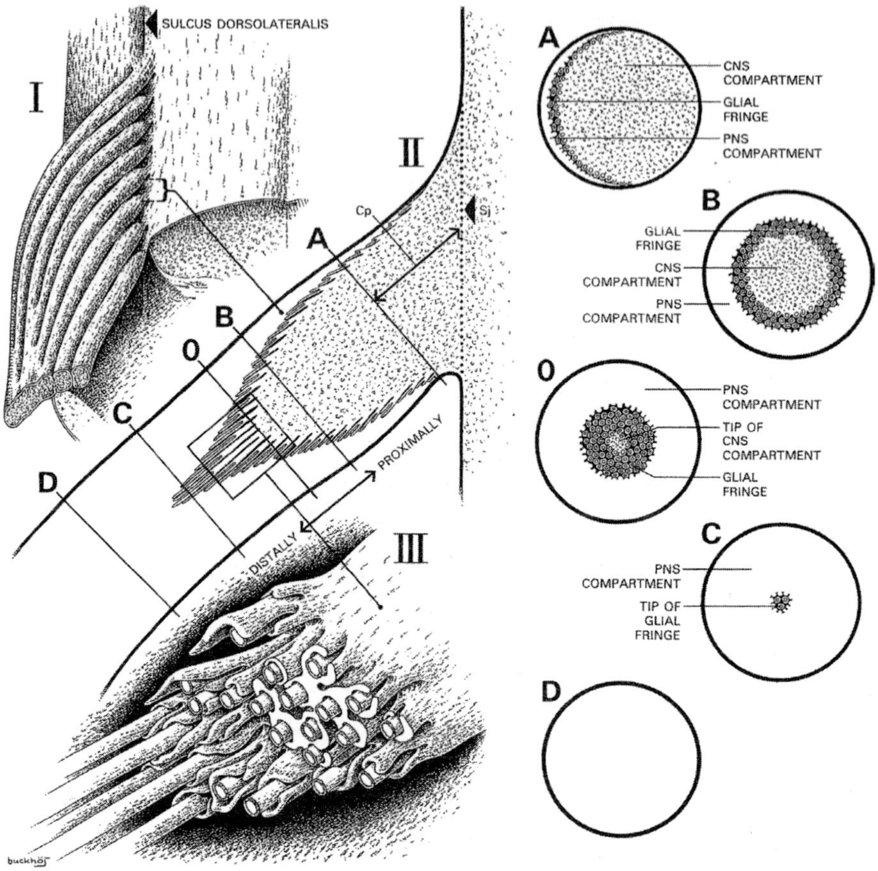

Fig. 2 Schematic drawings showing (I) the S1 dorsal root, (II) a frontal section through the transitional region of an S1 doorsal rootlet, and (III) the distal part of the glial fringe. (**I**) The dorsal root S1 and part of its spinal cord segment as viewed from behind. The rootlet marked out by the bracket is present at higher magnification in (II). (**II**) Frontal section through the TR. The proximal and distal directions as well as the longitudinal axis of the rootlet are indicated. Five reference cross-section levels (A, B, C, D, and O) through the proximal part of the S1 dorsal rootlet are marked. The transitional region extends between levels A and C. The dotted line indicates the spinal cord–rootlet junction (Sj). The wedge-shaped part of the rootlet situated between level A and the spinal cord–rootlet junction (Sj) is denoted the connecting piece (Cp). The tip of the cone-shaped CNS compartment is situated at level O. The tip of the glial fringe is located at level C. Level D runs through the stereotype part of the rootlet some 200–400 μm distal to the TR. The picture is not drawn to scale. (**III**) Artistic view of glial fringe. Only myelinated fibres are indicated (from Carlstedt 1977).

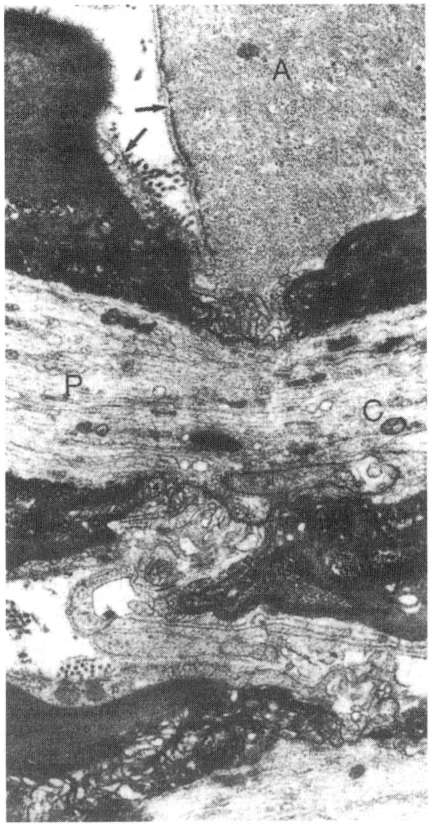

Fig. 3 Electron micrograph of a longitudinal section through a transitional node of Ranvier. The proximal end of part of the glial fringe surrounding the proximal peripheral paranode is seen outside the node gap. The Schwann cell basement membrane is continuous with that outlining the astrocyte outside the node gap (×25 000) (from Berthold and Carlstedt 1977).

redistribution of the thinnest nerve fibres to the surface of the rootlet is the anatomical basis for superficial rhizotomy as pain treatment (Sindou *et al.* 1974). The myelinated fibres change from a PNS to a CNS type of organisation in a transitional node of Ranvier situated at the proximal end of a glial fringe cul-de-sac. This is a hybrid PNS–CNS node of Ranvier (Fig. 3).

The outline of the CNS part of the root is most irregular. The Schwann cell basement membrane is at the bottom of the various

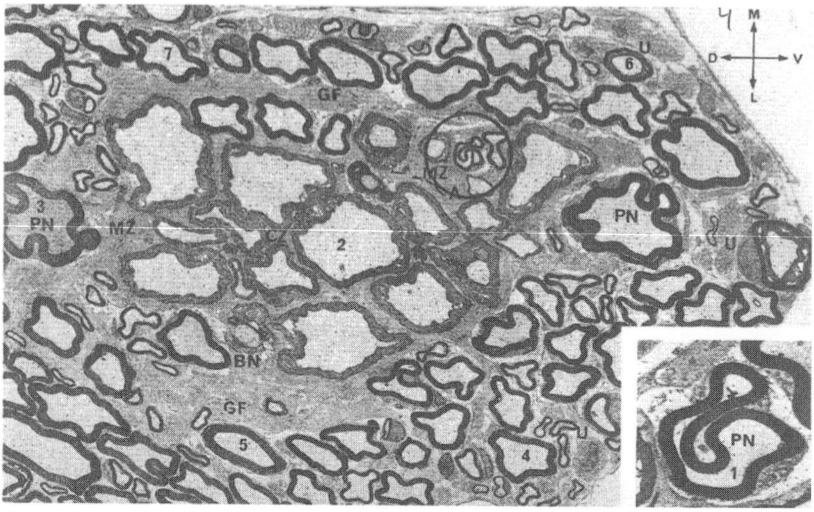

Fig. 4 Electron micrograph of cross-section (700 A thick) through the midpart of the TR in cat S1 dorsal root. The PNS is surrounding the CNS part of the root. Most large myelinated fibres are of CNS type and are localised to the centre of the picture. The main part of the smaller fibres are in the outer zone of the root and are of PNS type. Note the high occurrence of unmyelinated fibres in the most superficial zone of the root. There are no vessels in the CNS part of the root. The orientation of the root is given by the reference directions MLDV, medial, lateral, dorsal, and ventral (×1500) (from Carlstedt 1977).

glial fringe cul-de-sac formations continuous with the glia limitans basement membrane coating the CNS part of the root and the glial fringe. At the bottom of a glial fringe cul-de-sac where the nerve fibres translate from the PNS to the CNS parts of the root, there is a unique apposition between astrocytes and Schwann cells, establishing direct contact between cells of the PNS and of the CNS (Fig. 3).

There is no distinct PNS–CNS structural borderline. The interface between the PNS and the CNS could be more of a chemical border based on contact inhibition, which as such prevents the "invasion" of one into the other, e.g. Schwann cells creeping into the spinal cord. Such situations occur only in experimental conditions, such as after irradiation damage to the root spinal cord junction (Sims and Gilmore 1983).

Degeneration and Regeneration

The response to injury is quite different in the PNS and the CNS parts of the root. The Schwann cells multiply and arrange themselves in longitudinal bands (known as Bugner), acting as scaffolds to support and guide the new and growing axons. In the CNS part of the root, on the other hand, the preinjury structure of astrocytic channels surrounding the first part of the nerve fibres as they pass into the spinal cord is deranged. The central nervous glial cells, mainly astrocytes, proliferate and form an unpermissive gliotic outgrowth, a glial scar (Reier *et al.* 1983). The mechanical stress from root traction injury appears to enhance proliferation and migration of astrocytes into the PNS part of the root. Mechanical stress on the TR, as it would occur in a traction injury to the plexus, provokes a vigorous outgrowth of astrocytic processes (Nomura *et al.* 2002). Tissue components of the PNS part of the root, such as neurotrophic factors and extracellular matrix molecules, support nerve fibre regrowth, but these elements are not present in the CNS (Korsching 1993). Structural and chemical differences are of importance for the reactions to injury.

The anatomy of the spinal nerve root makes the TR a most attractive model for studies of injury-induced reactions of nerve fibres and glial cells, both in the PNS and in the CNS. It is possible to manipulate the nerve fibres distally in the PNS part of the root, without interfering with the integrity and vascular system of the CNS tissue in the proximal part of the root (Berthold *et al.* 1993). A lesion in the distal part of the dorsal root is remote from the CNS tissue, but it will lead to anterograde axonal degeneration in the PNS and CNS parts of the same nerve fibres. No mechanical or indirect vascular trauma is caused to the CNS root segment. This region has attracted a lot of interest as an injury model in studies of regeneration strategies to promote regrowth after a spinal cord injury. It is easily accessible and clearly delineated. Moreover, it offers an opportunity to avoid direct CNS damage, which is virtually impossible in studies on spinal cord tracts; allows us to compare regeneration in grey and white matters; and allows us to analyse the behaviour of the regenerating terminals, both structurally and with electrophysiology.

In the adult mammal, injured neurons cannot negotiate an elongation across the TR into or out of the spinal cord without manipulations and the influence of molecular or cellular supplements (see below) (Oorschot and Jones 1990). The astrocytic barrier, developed as a response to nerve fibre degeneration, is most effective in preventing regeneration. Several axons are arrested, forming terminal enlargements or synaptoid endings indicating contact inhibition (Fig. 5) (Carlstedt 1985a). Different types of nerve cells — some of which are known to have regenerative capacity within the CNS environment, such as cholinergic, catecholaminergic, and embryonic neurons — are unable to cross the TR when transplanted to the dorsal root (Carlstedt 1995; Carlstedt 1997). However, regeneration is possible in the very immature animal, before an astrocyte-rich TR has been developed (Carlstedt 1997). After injury in such animals, there is regrowth into the grey matter of the local spinal cord

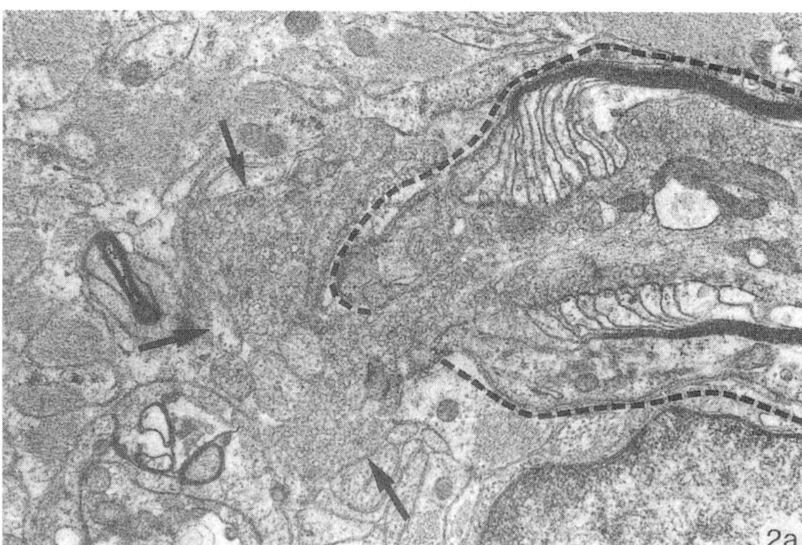

Fig. 5 Electromicrograph of longitudinal section through the TR after injury: the terminal part of a nerve fibre at the PNS–CNS interface. The axon emerges from the PNS type of myelin sheath in a seminode of Ranvier, before swelling and forming a terminal (arrows) filled with round agranular vesicles (×25 000) (from Carlstedt *et al.* 1989).

segment as well, along the fibre tracts (Carlstedt 1988). From that lesson, a strategy to promote PNS–CNS regeneration was developed, basically to delete the TR and to introduce or reimplant the root back into the spinal cord (Fig. 6).

After a detached dorsal root was reimplanted into the spinal cord, there was some abortive growth of dorsal root fibres into the spinal

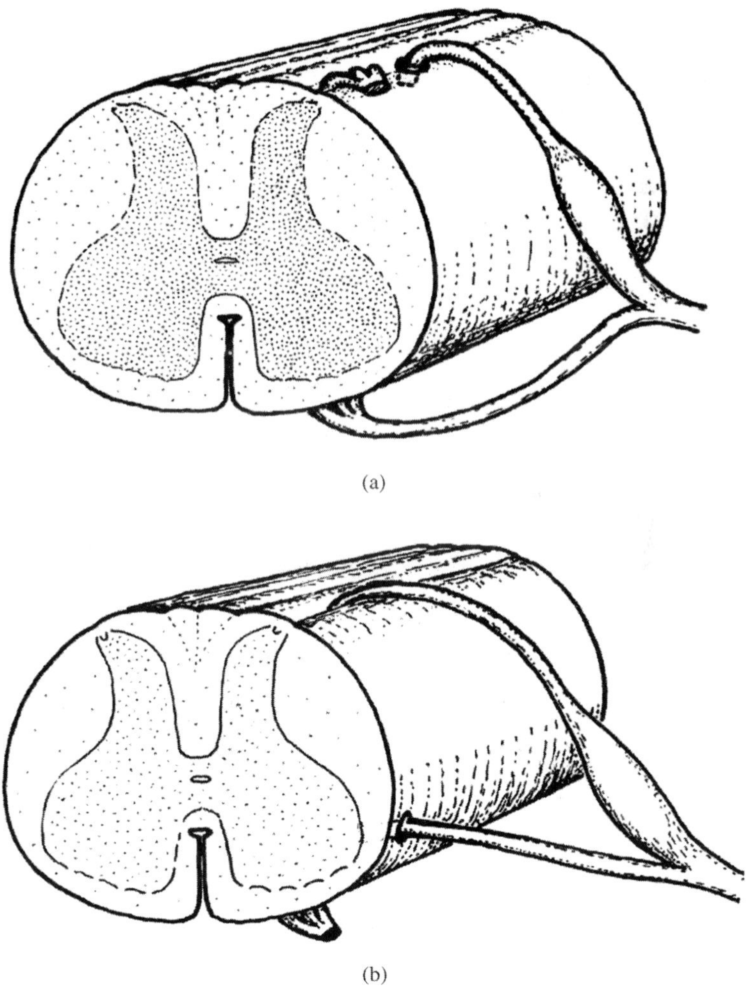

Fig. 6 Schematic drawings on implantation strategies for (a) dorsal and (b) ventral roots after the TR has been deleted.

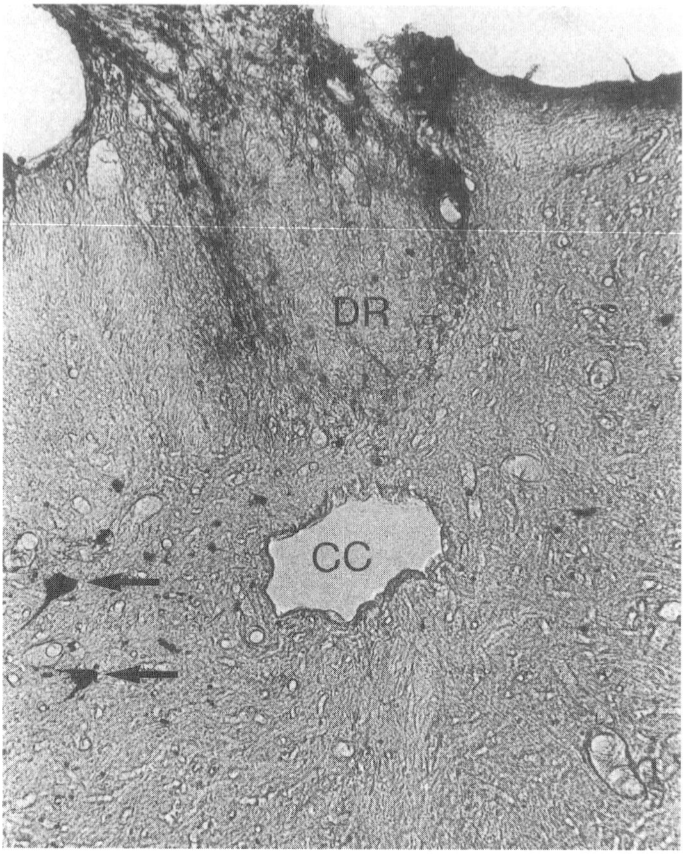

Fig. 7 Light micrograph of cross-section through the site of dorsal root (DR) implantation into the dorsal part of the spinal cord. HRP-labelled spinal cord neurons (arrows) are seen to the left of the central canal (CC) (×180) (from Carlstedt 1985b).

cord and, more importantly, a substantial outgrowth of dorsal horn neurons to the injured dorsal root (Fig. 7) (Carlstedt 1997). The potential of dorsal horn, or secondary, sensory neurons to elongate peripherally into the growth-promoting PNS tissue was further augmented by deleting the dorsal root ganglion, and in this way allowing for more "space" or Schwann cell columns to receive outgrowing axons. By this surgery, nerve cells intrinsic to the spinal cord had demonstrated an ability to grow also in the PNS. In double-labelling

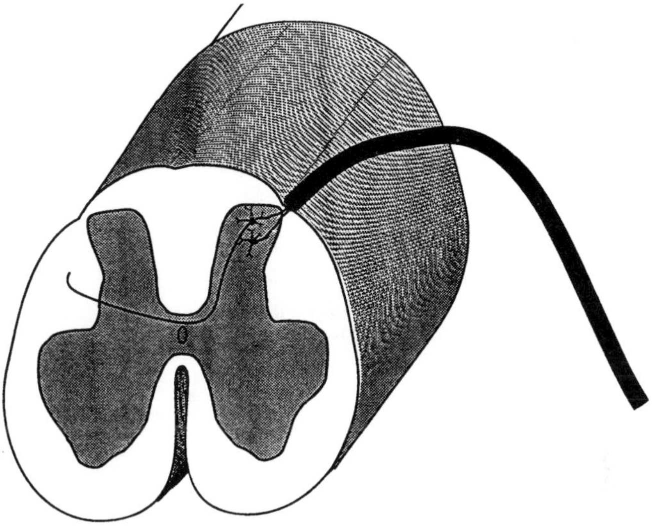

Fig. 8 Summary diagram of principal types of labelled neurons in the dorsal horn after dorsal root ganglionectomy and implantation. Dorsal horn neurons send extensions along the implanted dorsal root and retain their projections within the CNS (Carlstedt *et al.* 1991).

experiments, it was possible to demonstrate that such dorsal horn neurons had retained their rostral connections (Fig. 8) (Carlstedt *et al.* 1991). In effect, dorsal horn nerve cells had replaced the dorsal root ganglion cells and re-established connectivity between the spinal cord and the periphery. Any functional consequences of this surgery have not yet been demonstrated when applied to humans. This strategy was also experimentally applied to the ventral root injuries with immediate convincing functional outcome (see Chap. 8).

Regrowth into the spinal cord after dorsal root lesion was demonstrated when growth was augmented by transplantation of glial cells (Kliot *et al.* 1990), conditioning lesions (Chong *et al.* 1999), or neurotrophic factors (Ramer *et al.* 2000), as well as by transplantation using olfactory ensheathing cells (OECs) (Ramon-Cueto and Nieto-Sampedro 1994). For various reasons, such as conflicting outcome in different laboratories, particularly regarding the outcome from transplantation of OECs, these strategies have not yet been translated into clinical and human treatment.

Transplantation of OECs was known to induce regeneration and recovery in spinal cord lesions mainly by establishing a pathway (Li *et al.* 1997). The same protocol was used in dorsal root injury. After OECs were applied to the cut end of a dorsal root and the root was reopposed to the spinal cord, ingrowth of dorsal root fibres into the spinal cord occurred (Li *et al.* 2004). An interposition of OECs between the Schwann cells and the astrocytes induced "bridging channels" from the PNS to the CNS parts of the root, which allowed dorsal root nerve fibres to enter the spinal cord (Li *et al.* 2004). This arrangement appears similar to the native arrangement at the TR of Schwann cell columns surrounding individual nerve fibres in the channels of the astrocytic fringe (see above). Regenerated nerve fibres could be demonstrated within the dorsal horn as well as within the white matter of the dorsal columns. There seems to be a unique ability of the OECs to reconstruct pathways along which axons can grow. There is obviously a potential clinical application in the use of these cells in the repair of avulsed dorsal roots.

The basic requirements for the regeneration of function after a spinal nerve root avulsion injury are the survival of nerve cells situated close to the injury, and the regrowth along a trajectory of new nerve fibres consisting of CNS growth-inhibitory tissue in the spinal cord and PNS growth-promoting tissue in nerves.

A proximal nerve plexus injury means a high risk of degeneration and death to both sensory as well as motor nerve cells. A lesion close to the dorsal root ganglion provokes apoptotic death of the primary sensory neurons in the dorsal root ganglion, particularly small-diameter neurons connected to the skin (Hu and McLachlan 2003). Studies of molecular changes in the injured brachial plexus may identify substances that can curtail nerve cell death, as well as be of value when trying to identify new treatments to enhance repair. Dorsal root ganglions were obtained from patients during standard brachial plexus repairs following trauma, causing root avulsion injuries. By using this tissue, it was possible for the first time in man, and in any other species, to quantify and localise the glial cell line–derived neurotrophic factor (GDNF) and its receptor component Ret in dorsal root ganglion neurons (DRGNs) after avulsion injury. It was found that, in man, after brachial plexus avulsion injury, GDNF — trophic to sensory and motor neurons — is upregulated in medium- and small-sized DRGNs (Bar *et al.* 1998). Significantly higher levels of GDNFs were found in avulsed DRGNs than in control postmortem ganglion. This is likely to reflect an increase of GDNF uptake and transport to the cell body by the sensory neurons, as satellite or Schwann cells contained high levels of GDNF. Its receptor Ret was not affected by the avulsion (Fig. 9). The increased production of GDNF in satellite cells in the DRG could have a paracrine trophic role in DRGNs.

Shortly after the injury, there was a remarkable increase in interleukin-6 (IL-6), which is a member of the neuropoietic cytokine family (Saldanha *et al.* 2000). IL-6 and its receptor are required for nerve regeneration. The acute increase of IL-6 could originate from sensory cell bodies themselves or from inflammatory cells. This increase may have autocrine or paracrine effects, which may aid cell survival or have a role in nerve fibre sprouting and regrowth. The upregulation of these neurotrophic factors in DRGNs, most important after avulsion injury, suggests that GDNF as well as IL-6, which support the survival of peripheral and central neurons, may play a role in injured human sensory ganglia. There is a potential therapeutic role for locally applied recombinant human GDNFand IL-6 in human nerve repair.

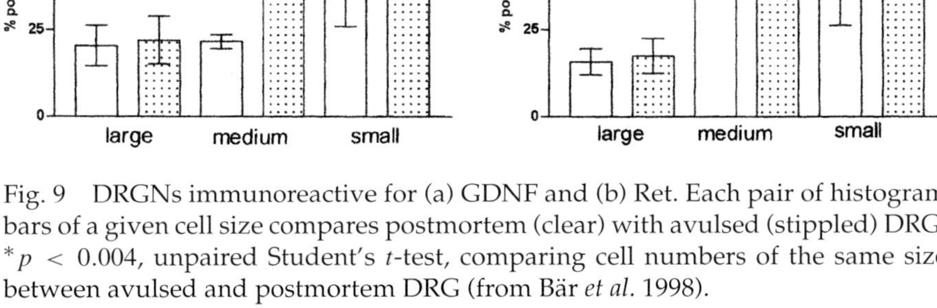

Fig. 9 DRGNs immunoreactive for (a) GDNF and (b) Ret. Each pair of histogram bars of a given cell size compares postmortem (clear) with avulsed (stippled) DRG. $*p < 0.004$, unpaired Student's *t*-test, comparing cell numbers of the same size between avulsed and postmortem DRG (from Bär *et al.* 1998).

Death of dorsal horn neurons results directly from the trauma of dorsal root avulsion or transganglionically through the loss of nerve terminals in the dorsal horn. The effect of dorsal root avulsion is devastating, compared to root section or rhizotomy, as described in laboratory experiments (Zhao *et al.* 1998). The disappearance of sensory neurons triggers changes in connectivity in the dorsal horn, leading to abnormal signalling (Mannion and Woolf 2000). This is believed to be some of the pathophysiological background to the classical and typical pain affecting patients with severe brachial plexus injury (Ovelmen-Levitt 1988; Berman *et al.* 1998).

Motoneurons are rapidly killed by ventral root avulsion (Koliatsos *et al.* 1994). Disconnection from the periphery means that interrupted supply of neutrotrophic factors, together with vascular trauma leading to excitotoxicity, drastically reduces the number of motoneurons up to about 90% of the normal population (Lindå *et al.* 1993; Koliatsos *et al.* 1994). Other mechanisms to motoneuron death, such as an inflammatory response to avulsion by means of microglial activation from cytokines, have also been described (Olsson *et al.* 2000). Already 2 weeks after injury, about half of all motoneurons in the pertinent spinal cord segment have disappeared. There is further neuronal death over time (Bergerot *et al.* 2004). A swift intervention to re-establish contact between the injured nerve cells and the periphery with its supply of neurotrophic substances would counteract nerve cell loss in these injuries.

The early response to avulsion in motoneurons means a shrinkage in the size of the soma and dendrites. The number of synaptic connections with the injured neuron is diminished, especially on the cell body and proximal dendrites. There is a preferential loss of excitatory inputs to the motoneuron in this situation, probably leaving the cells under an inhibitory influence during the repair process (Lindå *et al.* 1992). These events mirror a shift in the metabolism of the severed motoneurons from subserving the role for the motoneuron as a commander of motor activity to a state where the primary goal is to survive and produce new axons. This is reflected in an increase in the mRNA expression of proteins associated with cell survival, including growth factors such as BDNF and receptors (Piehl *et al.*

1998), and proteins for axonal growth including GAP-43 (Lindå *et al.* 1992). Motoneurons that are rescued by connection to a reimplanted ventral root, for instance, or by a peripheral nerve graft seem to be very potent in producing new axons. One motoneuron can produce several myelinated axon-like processes; in some cases, such projections emerge from a dendrite — known as dendraxons (Lindå *et al.* 1985) — rather than from the nerve cell body.

The recent developments and gains in knowledge from studies of molecular biology have demonstrated the importance of the timing of repair of nerve injuries. Already 1 month after injury, the expressions of growth factors and their receptors have declined to the extent that the outcome of repair is less favourable than if it is done immediately after the injury (for a review, see Gordon *et al.* 2003). With regard to root avulsion injury, time-dependent neuron death adds to the urgency in reconstructing these injuries, as reimplanting the avulsed ventral root to some extent maintains the population of spinal cord motoneurons (Carlstedt *et al.* 1993). Rescue of motoneurons after ventral root avulsion has been described after growth-inducing or neurotrophic substances, such as BDNF and GDNF, were given to experimental animals (Li *et al.* 1995; Novikov *et al.* 1997). However, the application of such molecules seems to have little effect on the restoration of function and could in fact be counterproductive, as reported regarding lesions to the peripheral nerve (Gordon *et al.* 2003).

In a recent study, the combination of the growth factor GDNF and the neuroprotective drug riluzole drastically improved function in animal experiments. In an already reduced population of motoneurons, combined treatment with such substances caused an augmentation in the production of new processes, which increased functional outcome (Fig. 10) (Bergerot *et al.* 2004). It was demonstrated that immediate treatment involving surgical reimplantation of avulsed ventral root, intrathecal GDNF delivery, or intraperitoneal injection of riluzole for 2 weeks ameliorates motoneuron death to 80% of control; but the combination of the different treatment paradigms did not further enhance survival, except when GDNF was combined with ventral root implantation, as assessed

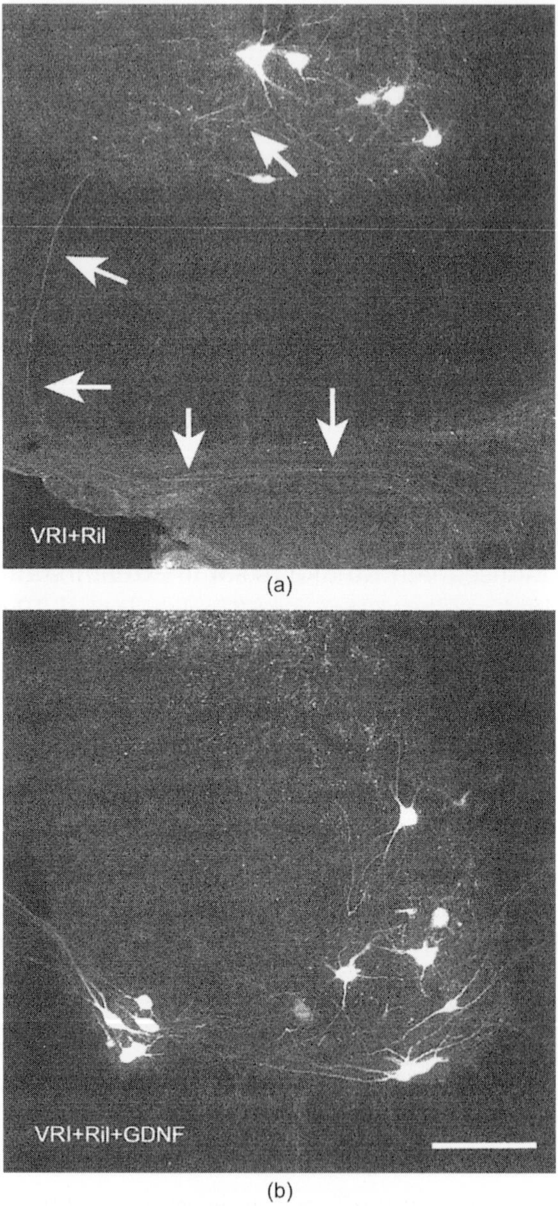

Fig. 10 Examples of enhanced growth of processes from motoneurons after avulsion and implantation of ventral roots in animals treated with (a) riluzole or (b) riluzole and GDNF. Some axons can be seen entering the implanted ventral root (arrows). Scale bar = 200 μm (from Bergerot *et al.* 2004).

after 2 weeks. At 3 months follow-up, the neuroprotective effect of reimplantation (80%) was not maintained unless it was combined with riluzole and GDNF treatment (Fig. 11). Analysis of regenerating motoneurons showed that riluzole increased the number of dendrites per motoneuron as a sign of more robust regeneration (Fig. 10). Using two different locomotor tests, it was found that significant functional recovery approaching normal values occurred only after reimplantation of avulsed ventral roots, together with GDNF and riluzole treatment (Fig. 12).

These results show that functional recovery is correlated to enhanced dendritic complexity and increased survival of motoneurons. Riluzole promotes dendritic outgrowth, and neurotrophins such as GDNF promote motoneuron survival and axonal regeneration; both are required for functional recovery, possibly by increasing neurotransmitter levels or synthesis in motoneurons. A combination of substances that provokes such neuronal reactions is needed

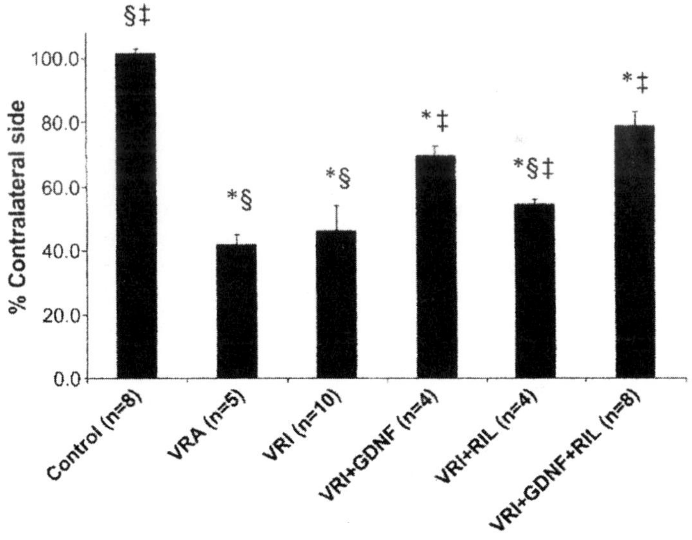

Fig. 11 Quantitative analysis of motoneuron cell survival in different treatment groups 3 months after avulsion injury. ANOVA followed by post hoc analysis showed the following interactions: $*$ means significantly different from control, ‡ means significantly different from VRA, and § means significantly different from VRI + GDNF + RIL ($P < 0.05$) (from Bergerot *et al.* 2004).

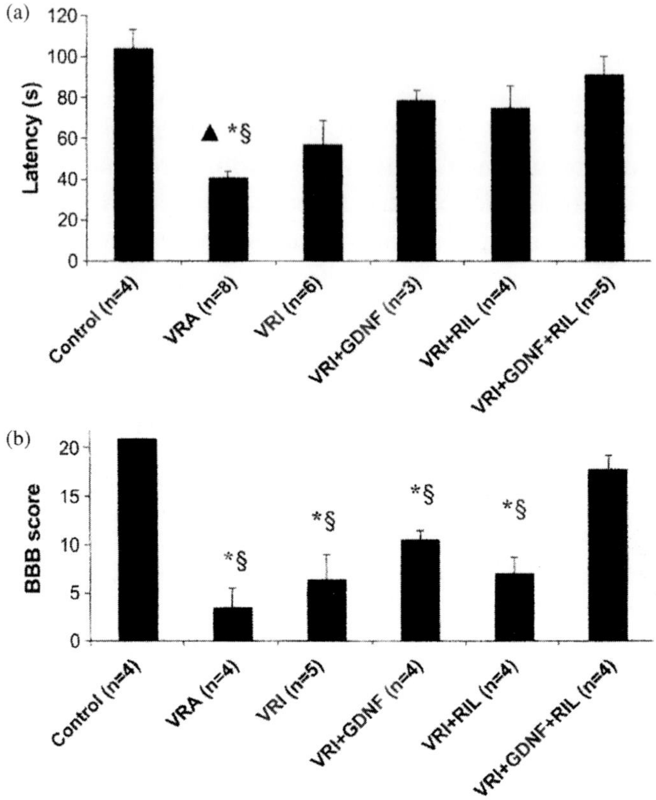

Fig. 12 Analysis of locomotor ability using (a) rotarod test and (b) BBB locomotor rating scale. Post hoc analysis showed groups that were significantly different from control (∗), VRI + GDNF (▲), or VRI + GDNF + RIL (§). Note that VRI + GDNF + RIL was significantly different from the VRA group in both tests, while it was not significantly different from the control in either test (from Bergerot *et al.* 2004).

to achieve a good outcome from the repair of root avulsion injury. Thus, combination treatment may offer a new therapeutic strategy for treating patients with avulsion injury.

In separate experiments, the delivery of neurotrophins to the injured motoneurons was made more concentrated and sustained over a longer period of time by means of gene transfer with adeno-associated viral (AAV) vectors encoding GDNF and BDNF (Fig. 13). There was an overexpression of these factors in the motoneuron pool after extensive ventral root avulsion for 16 weeks. There was very

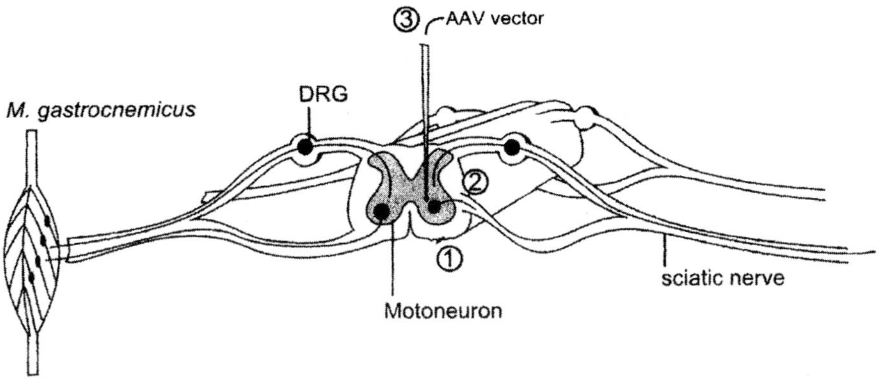

Fig. 13 Overview of the experiment. Lumbar ventral roots (L2–L6) were avulsed (1), thereby disconnecting muscles in the hind limb from motor input through the sciatic nerve. To introduce a growth terrain for the injured motoneurons to regrow its connections, the L4 root was reimplanted (2). To promote survival of injured motoneurons, AAV vectors encoding BDNF or GDNF were injected towards the injured neuron pool (3). The hind limbs of experimental animals were then tested functionally during the experiment period (1 and 4 months postinjury). The number of ChAT-positive fibres was determined in the sciatic nerve, and retrograde tracing with FB was performed to recognise cells in the spinal cord that had regrown their neurites in the sciatic nerve. DRG = dorsal root ganglion (from Blits *et al.* 2004).

little recovery of function, however, as the high concentration of the neurotrophins in the motoneuron pool prevented an elongation into the reimplanted ventral root and, rather, caused the formation of a local network of motoneuron axons restricted to the ventral horn (Fig. 14). The level of neurotrophic factors within the ventral horn obviously promoted sprouting, but prevented directional growth of the new motoneuron axons (Blits *et al.* 2004).

The spinal root avulsion injury is a type of spinal cord lesion that has a longitudinal direction rather than a transverse course, as in the classical spinal cord lesions. Regrowth of new axons after such a longitudinal spinal cord injury must therefore occur in the spinal cord (Fig. 15). A remarkable ability to regenerate and elongate was noted after a discrete lesion of the central part of motoneuron axons was produced in the ventral funiculus of the spinal cord (Risling *et al.* 1983). The potency of motoneuron regeneration after an intramedullary injury is illustrated by the fact that lesioned

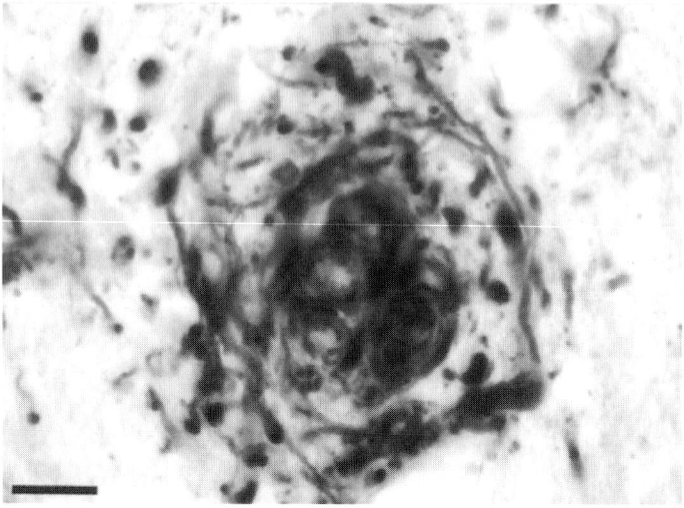

Fig. 14 Labyrinth of ChAT-positive motoneuron fibres in the ventral horn after avulsion and reimplantation of ventral root in animal 4 months after transduction with AAV vector encoding the BDNF gene. Scale bar = 100 μm (from Blits *et al.* 2004).

motoneurons can produce more than one myelinating axon-like process through the lesion area; in some cases, such axons may derive from distal dendrites known as dendraxons (Lindå *et al.* 1985). This regenerative capacity was explored after ventral root avulsion in a long series of animal experiments. The avulsed ventral root was reimplanted into the ventral part of the spinal cord as close as possible to the site of avulsion.

It became obvious from intracellular staining experiments after ventral root reimplantation that motoneuron axon regeneration occurred among CNS glial cells, astrocytes, and oligodendrocytes (Fig. 16). The new motoneuron axons had been myelinated by oligodendrocytes. The most central intramedullary part of the new motoneuron axons exhibit all of the characteristics of a CNS fibre, i.e. CNS-type myelin sheaths interrupted by CNS-type nodes of Ranvier (Fig. 16). As the first part of the axons had regenerated for a considerable distance with the spinal cord before entering the root, implantation into the cord not necessary had to be deep, but just below the

Ventral root reimplantation

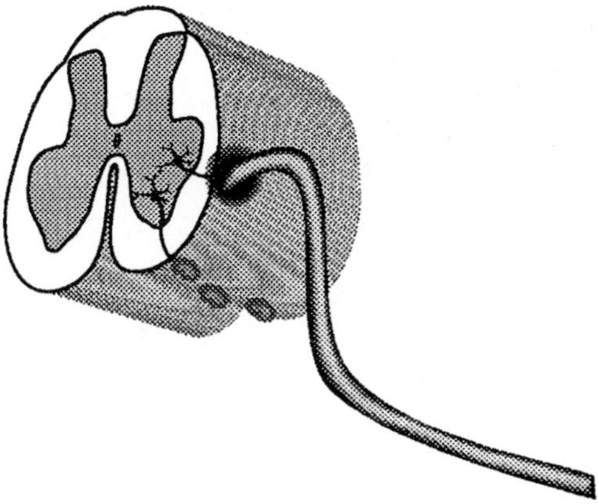

Fig. 15 Schematic drawing illustrating the location of scar tissue and regeneration of motoneuron axons within the spinal cord segment after ventral root avulsion and reimplantation into the ventrolateral aspect of the spinal cord (from Risling *et al.* 1993).

surface of the spinal cord (Fig. 15). Introducing the avulsed root or a PNS transplant deep to a cut in the pia–glial membrane is of course less dangerous or less harmful to local neurons and long fibre tracts, probably with few negative functional consequences (see below in humans).

The mechanism supporting the initial CNS regeneration of the motoneuron axons within the spinal cord is not fully understood. A promoting factor of obvious potential is the denervated PNS tissue in the ventral root just outside the lesion area. Still, a regrowing motoneuron axon must negotiate elongation through the CNS tissue of the spinal cord. There is a region of scarring, caused by the avulsion and reimplantation, to pass before the growth-promoting PNS tissue is reached. However, there are particular conditions in the scar tissue, as well as within the motoneuron itself, that promote this spinal cord regeneration.

Although generally considered abortive, it is obvious that regeneration within the spinal cord, particularly its grey substance, can occur in some situations, e.g. after lesions in the immature animal

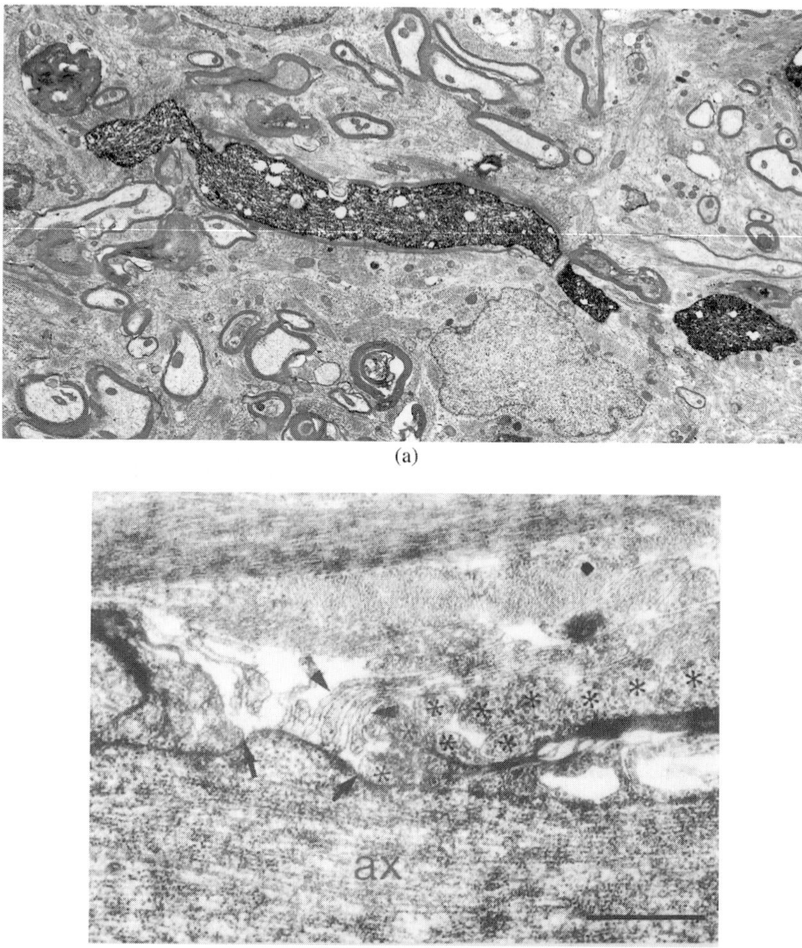

Fig. 16 Electron micrograph of HRP-labelled motoneuron axon regrowing within the spinal cord after ventral root avulsion and reimplantation. (a) The axon has regenerated through the CNS tissue and is surrounded by CNS glial cells (×2500). (b) CNS-type nodes of Ranvier in the same fibre (×25 000).

or by means of transplantation of immature neurons, specifically cholinergic and cathecolaminergic neurons (Wictorin and Björklund 1992). Compensatory growth, such as collateral sprouting by dorsal horn neurons after dorsal root injury (Murray and Goldberger 1968) and the growth of supernumerary axons from motoneurons after peripheral nerve lesions (Havtorn and Kellerth 1987) are other examples of neuronal growth in the spinal cord.

Motoneuron axons regrow from the ventral horn through scar tissue composed of a trabecular framework of astrocyte processes and leptomeningeal cells as well as phagocytic and inflammatory cells. This scar is surrounded by an expanded extracellular space containing numerous collagen fibres (Risling *et al.* 1983). There is no regrowth through intact white matter. It is known that axon growth depends on the presence of extracellular matrix molecules with adhesive properties. The lesion area after root avulsion contains a number of such molecules, for example laminin, tenascin, and various types of collagen, often arranged in tubular formations in which new outgrowing axons can occur (Risling *et al.* 1993; Frisen *et al.* 1994; Frisen *et al.* 1995). After avulsion, there is an increased expression of insulin-like growth factor (IGF) binding protein 6 (IGFBP-6) in the injured motoneurons. The scar in the spinal cord expresses IGF-1, which will thus be available for and possibly mediate trophic effects on the injured motoneurons (Hammarberg *et al.* 1998).

There is a clear dominance of astrocytes with signs of mitotic activity in the scar, but there are very few oligodendrocytes, even shortly after the trauma. It should be noted that new astrocytes can be generated from the ependymal stem cells after a spinal cord injury (Johansson *et al.* 1999). The new and reactive astrocytes express receptors for neurotrophin substances (Frisen *et al.* 1992; Frisen *et al.* 1993) that obviously can bind the neurotrophins and present to the growing motoneuron axon those which are of importance in the process of regeneration. An unusually rapid elimination of oligodendrocytes occurs, leaving only about 5% one week after avulsion compared with about 60% in the naive ventral funiculus. A much slower elimination of oligodendrocytes from lack of axonal contact occurs during the Wallerian degeneration of spinal cord tracts (Fransson 1985). The rapid death of oligodendrocytes may be of relevance for the observed regenerative response, as CNS myelin and the myelinating cell, the oligodendrocyte, have been reported to impede the regrowth of axons (Schwab and Caroni 1988).

The repulsive substances belonging to the semaphorin family, best known for their capacity to repel axonal outgrowth, are found in central nervous scars (Pasterkamp *et al.* 1998). Such substances were also found in the spinal cord avulsion scar and in injured motoneurons (Lindholm *et al.* 2004). Of interest was the discovery that the vascular endothelial growth factor (VEGF) — which has an important angiogenic effect, but is also neuroprotective and important in the process of growth and repair, particularly for motoneurons in the spinal cord (Oosthuyse *et al.* 2001) — shares the same receptor, neuropilin-1 (Soker *et al.* 1998). A possible competition between these two substances for the receptor could curtail the repulsive function of semaphorin in the avulsion scar. A recent finding of the promotion of VEGF production in motoneurons by a hypoxia inducible factor (HIF) protein (Sköld *et al.* 2004) further explains the complicated cascade of events that follows avulsion injury and that makes it possible for spinal cord motoneurons to produce spinal cord regeneration.

There exists a long-standing (years) defect in the blood–brain barrier, which is unique compared with other types of spinal cord injuries (weeks). Such a defect allows blood-borne substances of importance for regeneration as well as cells such as macrophages and T-cells to enter the scar tissue together with other blood-borne substances that stimulate nerve growth and are normally excluded from nerve tissue. Obviously, the scar that develops in the spinal cord after root avulsion is different from other scars in the CNS, with a unique content of several tissue components and substances characteristic of the peripheral nerve, rather than the spinal cord, that are crucial for regeneration. These details are certainly of importance in promoting the spinal cord regrowth of injured motoneurons.

New axons leave the spinal cord through the implanted ventral roots. In the newly established posttraumatic TR, there was no sign of Schwann cells entering the spinal cord from the implanted root, but numerous glial cell processes were found in the proximal part of the implanted ventral root. Some fibres that were unmyelinated in the spinal cord were myelinated by Schwann cells in the root (cf. Carlstedt 1977). Larger fibres were invested by CNS myelin proximal to the TR and by Schwann cell-produced myelin in the root.

Regenerated Function

The initial experiments that showed restitution of muscle function after the reimplantation of avulsed ventral roots into the spinal cord (Carlstedt *et al.* 1986) (Fig. 17) were later confirmed in many laboratories (Horvat *et al.* 1987; Hoffman *et al.* 1990; Smith and Kodama 1991; Bertelli and Mira 1994). However, those were crude experiments which could not demonstrate with certainty that a specific injured or axonotomised motoneuron had regenerated function, as there are several possibilities of false-positive results from anastomoses or collaterals from uninjured nerve cells. The crucial experiment in this, as well as in other studies of regeneration, is the demonstration that the same neurons give rise to function when groups or individual nerve cells are injured. Unfortunately, such studies are rare even in spinal cord injury research, leaving too much for biased speculation on "cure for paralysis".

After ventral root avulsion and reimplantation, a claim of restored function with certainty can only follow from intracellular experiments where the same motoneuron is examined by physiological techniques and then stained in order to be identified and

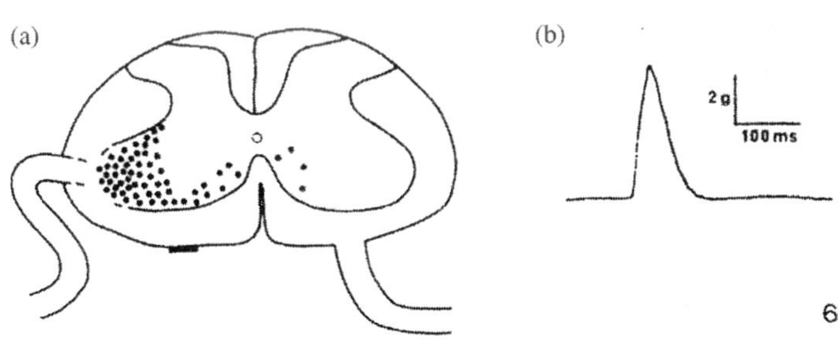

Fig. 17 (a) Transverse distribution of 6l retrogradely horseradish peroxidase (HRP)-labelled neurons in the L4 spinal cord segment in one rat 3 months after avulsion of the left ventral roots L3–L5 and implantation of root L3 in the L4 segment. Three days before the rat was killed, the sciatic nerve on the operated side was divided in the popliteal fossa and a cap with HRP solution was applied to the proximal stump. (b) Twitch response of the left triceps surae muscle after stimulation of the implanted ventral root L3 in one rat 8 months after avulsion of the left ventral roots L3–L5 and implantation of root L3 in the L4 segment (from Carlstedt *et al.* 1986).

anatomically assessed after the animal has been sacrificed. This was done after ventral root avulsion and reimplantation in cats, and demonstrated that alpha and probably also gamma motoneurons were able to reinnervate ventral root implants. The regenerated axons could conduct impulses (Fig. 18) (Cullheim *et al.* 1989). The regenerated neurons could be excited or inhibited by impulses in afferent, intact, and dorsal roots, and their contribution to elicit reflex activity was normal such that muscle twitch response was induced by stimulation of the implanted ventral root. Other routes of regrowth could be excluded in these experiments. An effect of this surgery is that the injured motoneurons are reintegrated in the local segmental spinal cord reflex circuits, and are able to regenerate and reinnervate muscle.

The concept of functional regeneration by motoneurons injured from root avulsion was applied and tested in a brachial plexus injury situation in primates (Carlstedt *et al.* 1993). The main outcome of these experiments was that the deficits in proximal arm function could be corrected into useful activity by reimplantation of the avulsed cervical ventral roots. Although full range of motion was observed, electromyography (EMG) showed reduced activity in previously denervated muscles at maximal voluntary contraction compared with the unaffected control side.

By subjecting nerve fibres reinnervating the biceps muscle in these primates to HRP staining procedure, the localisation of their neurons was revealed. There was a larger and more spread-out spinal population of neurons on the lesioned side where root implantation had been performed. In addition to an equally large population of labelled neurons related to the region of normal biceps innervation within the ventral horn on both the operated and control sides, there was an equally large number of labelled neurons diffusely located throughout the motoneuron pool on the operated side (Fig. 19). Different functional types of neurons were apparently attracted to extend processes into the implanted ventral root. As judged by their position in the ventral horn, neurons that normally innervate trunk muscles, situated medially in the horn, contributed to the reinnervation of the biceps muscle. Also, cells

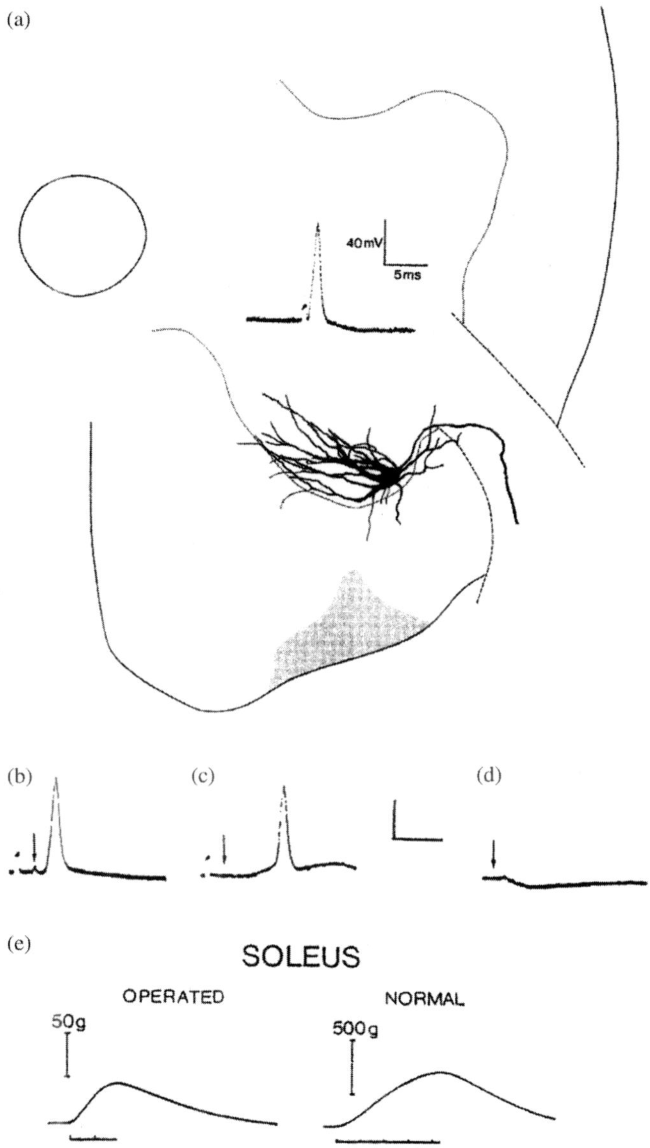

Fig. 18

normally supplying antagonistic muscles, such as triceps neurons, participated in the regeneration process to the biceps muscle. These experiments also revealed an alternative route to re-establish connectivity between the motoneuron pool and the avulsed roots. Abundant myelinated fibres could be followed from the avulsion site to the implanted root promoted by the matrix of the pia mater, which has a known competence for sustaining nerve fibre growth (Risling *et al.* 1993).

With regard to the ability of regenerating motoneurons to find the proper original muscle, results from rats and cats studies suggest that there occurred a substantial cross-innervation. For instance, reinnervation of the soleus muscle in the leg of a cat had occurred from neurons that, on stimulation, provoked an abnormal fast contraction, indicating that the reinnervating neuron is normally connected to fast-twitch muscles (Fig. 18). Functionally, this deficient directional specificity was correlated to both spactisity and cocontraction among agonistic and antagonistic muscles. In the primate experiments, ongoing motor unit activity in both the biceps and the triceps on the lesioned and operated sides were noted. During voluntary activation, it was not possible to achieve isolated contractions of

Fig. 18 (a) A cat spinal lumbar motoneuron visualized by intracellular staining with horseradish peroxidase. After avulsion and reimplantation of a ventral root laterally, a new axon has grown out into the implant. An action potential can be elicited by antidromic electrical stimulation of the ventral root. [(b)–(d)] Intracellular recordings from different motoneurons with axon outgrowth via implanted ventral roots. In (b) is shown an antidromically evoked action potential after stimulation of the implanted root. In (c), the same motoneuron has been orthodromically activated by stimulation of the tibial nerve in the popliteal fossa. In this way, an excitatory postsynaptic potential (EPSP) is produced via primary afferent fibres. The EPSP in turn elicits an action potential in yet another motoneuron. (d) An inhibitory postsynaptic potential (IPSP) is elicited after stimulation of the tibial nerve. Scale bars: vertical, 20 mV; horizontal, 2 ms. (e) Electrical stimulation of an implanted ventral root gives rise to a contraction in the soleus muscle. The much faster contraction time in the operated animal than in the normal one strongly suggests that reinnervating motoneurons normally support fast-twitch muscle fibres. Reproduced from Cullheim *et al.* (1999), with permission from Nature Publishing Group.

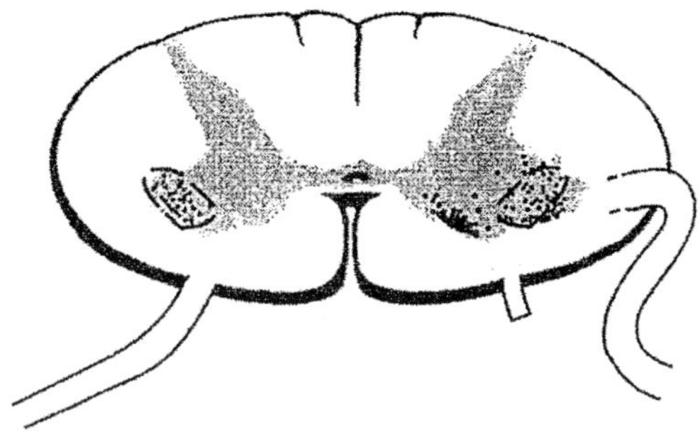

Fig. 19 Composite camera lucida drawing showing the distribution of HRP-labelled neurons (location not size-indicated) in the C6 spinal cord segment after injection of HRP in the biceps muscle on the operated and control sides. The hatched line indicates the normal region for biceps neurons. Note the abundance and diffuse occurrence of neurons with *de novo* formed connections with the biceps muscle on the operated side (from Hallin *et al.* 1999).

either biceps and the triceps without cocontraction of its antagonist (Fig. 20).

Several mechanisms can account for inappropriate reinnervation. Intraspinal reimplantation of avulsed ventral roots stimulated different types of ventral horn motoneurons to grow axons. Collateral sprouting, new aberrant axons (Havtorn and Kellerth 1987), and dendraxons (Lindå *et al.* 1985) from functionally different motoneurons could contribute to the reinnervation of a specific muscle. The new axons, when reaching the PNS conduit, elongated from the proximal part of the nerve trunk and had several possibilities to be sidetracked when encountering more distal branching points. In double-labelling experiments, simultaneous links to both antagonistic and agonistic muscles from the same neuron could not be demonstrated. The structural basis for deficient performance such as synkinesis or cocontraction was not due to the same neuron innervating antagonistic muscles, but rather was the effect of an unspecific reinnervation by inappropriate neurons under inappropriate supraspinal control.

The failing axonal guidance to correct targets could create a functional chaos, where attempted voluntary contraction would only result in uncoordinated mass muscle contractions. However, the

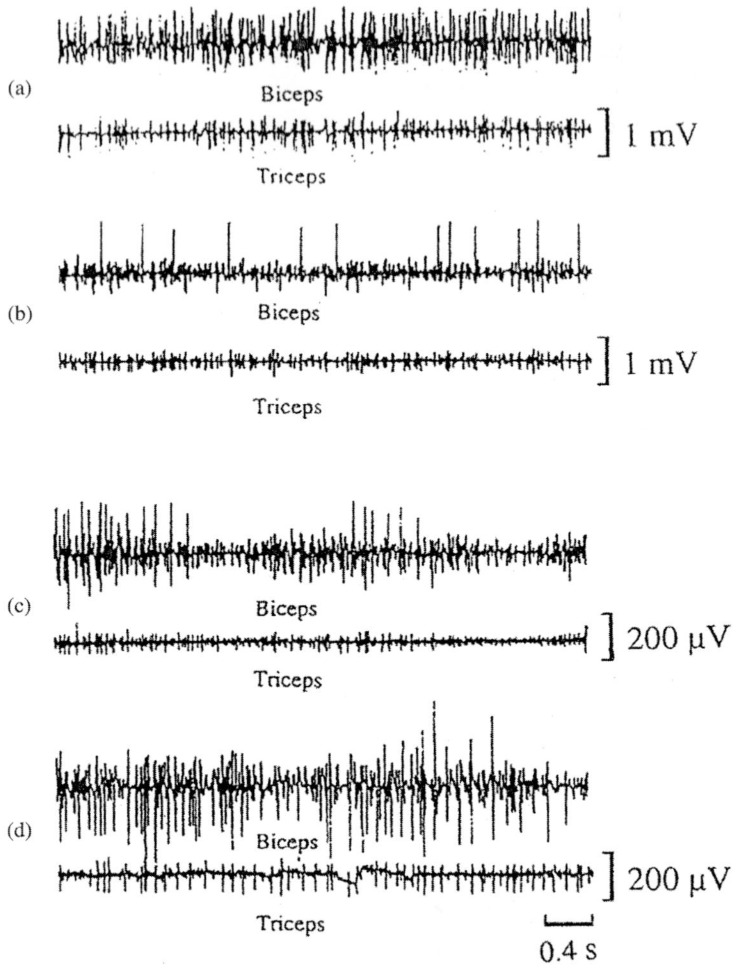

Fig. 20 Cocontraction in biceps and triceps muscles following ventral root avulsion from the spinal cord. Preparation where the C5–C7 ventral roots were reimplanted anterolaterally with 2 months delay are shown in (a) and (b); another totally denervated preparation is shown in (c) and (d). (a) Attempted preferential contraction of biceps muscle about 9 months after reinnervation accomplished by ventral root reimplantation with 2 months delay. (b) Attempted preferential contraction of triceps muscle. (c) Ongoing activity at rest in totally denervated preparation, i.e. where the C5–C8 ventral root contribution to the arm was totally avulsed but not reimplanted. (d) Attempted preferential biceps contraction in totally denervated preparation. Horizontal bar, 0.4 s; vertical bar, 1 mV [(a), (b)] and 200 μV [(c), (d)] (from Hallin *et al.* 1999).

initial muscle synkinesis from a random motoneuron–muscle reinnervation that initially disturbed function eventually developed into purposeful movements (Hallin *et al.* 1999; see also Chap. 8). Precision is achieved after injury and repair by the selective loss of inappropriate projections (pruning) over a period of time after the initial regeneration (Benett *et al.* 1986; MacKinnon *et al.* 1991). Deficient directional specificity during axonal elongation might eventually be corrected towards more functional specificity in the appropriate motor units, after establishing the initial nerve–muscle contact. A further consideration is the plasticity of motor centres, with reorganisation of motor cortex after the avulsion trauma (Kaas 1991).

Conclusion

The transitional region (TR) between the peripheral nervous system (PNS) and the central nervous system (CNS) is a highly specialised and unique part of the spinal nerve root, where regrowth of nerve fibres is arrested. Nerve fibre regeneration in between the spinal cord (CNS) and the spinal nerve roots (PNS) can occur when the TR is deleted. Superficial spinal cord implantation of severed roots just deep to the pia–glial membrane augments nerve cell survival and induces elongation of nerve fibres from the spinal cord to the nerves. Regenerated muscle activity occurs from root–spinal cord surgery. Nondirectional, unspecific motoneuron regeneration results in functional disturbances such as synkinesis and cocontractions.

References

Bar KJ, Saldanha GJF, Kennedy AJ *et al.*, GDNF and its receptor component Ret in injured human nerves and dorsal root ganglia, *Neuroreport* **9**:43–47, 1998.

Bennett MR, Ho S, Lavisdis NA, Competition between segmental nerves at end-plates in rat gastrocnemius muscle during loss of polyneuronal innervation, *J Physiol* **381**:351–376, 1986.

Bergerot A, Shortland PJ, Anand P *et al.*, Co-treatment with riluzole and GDNF is necessary for functional recovery after ventral root avulsion injury, *Exp Neurol* **187**:359–366, 2004.

Berman J, Birch R, Anand P, Pain following human brachial plexus injury with spinal cord root avulsion and the effect of surgery, *Pain* **75**:199–207, 1998.

Bertelli JA, Mira JC, Brachial plexus repair by peripheral nerve grafts directly into the spinal cord in rats: behavioural and anatomical evidence for functional recovery, *J Neurosurg* **81**:107–114, 1994.

Berthold CH, Carlstedt T, General organization of the transitional region in S1 dorsal rootlets, *Acta Physiol Scand Suppl* **446**:23–42, 1977.

Berthold CH, Carlstedt T, Corneliuson O, The central–peripheral transition zone, in Dyck PJ, Thomas PK, Griffin JW *et al.* (eds.), *Peripheral Neuropathy*, 3rd edn, Saunders, Philadelphia, PA, pp. 73–91, 1993.

Blits B, Carlstedt T, Ruitenberg MJ *et al.*, Rescue and sprouting of motoneurons following ventral root avulsion and reimplantation combined with intraspinal adeno-associated viral vector-mediated expression of glial cell line–derived neurotrophic factor or brain-derived neurotrophic factor, *Exp Neurol* **189**:303–316, 2004.

Carlstedt T, Observations on the morphology at the transition between the peripheral and the central nervous system in the cat, PhD thesis, Karolinska Institutet, Stockholm, Sweden, 1977.

Carlstedt T, Regenerating axons from nerve terminals at astrocytes, *Brain Res* **347**:188–191, 1985a.

Carlstedt T, Dorsal root innervation of spinal cord neurons after dorsal root implantation into the spinal cord of adult rats, *Neurosci Lett* **55**:343–348, 1985b.

Carlstedt T, Reinnervation of the mammalian spinal cord after neonatal dorsal root crush, *J Neurocytol* **17**:335–350, 1988.

Carlstedt T, Spinal nerve root injuries in brachial plexus lesions: basic science and clinical application of new surgical strategies. A review, *Microsurgery* **16**:13–16, 1995.

Carlstedt T, Nerve fibre regeneration across the peripheral–central transitional zone, *J Anat* **190**:51–56, 1997.

Carlstedt T, Aldskogius H, Rosario C, Extension of dorsal horn neurons into the severed and implanted dorsal root, *Restor Neurol Neurosci* **3**:205–209, 1991.

Carlstedt T, Cullheim S, Risling M, Ulfhake B, Nerve fibre regeneration across the PNS–CNS interface at the root–spinal cord junction, *Brain Res Bull* **22**:93–102, 1989.

Carlstedt T, Hallin RG, Hedstrom KG, Nilsson-Remahl IA, Functional recovery in primates with brachial plexus injury after spinal cord implantation of avulsed ventral roots, *J Neurol Neurosurg Psychiatr* **56**:649–654, 1993.

Carlstedt T, Lindå H, Cullheim S, Risling M, Reinnervation of hind limb muscles after ventral root avulsion and implantation in the lumbar spinal cord of the adult rat, *Acta Physiol Scand* **128**:645–646, 1986.

Chong MS, Woolf CJ, Haque NSK, Anderson PN, Axonal regeneration from injured dorsal roots into the spinal cord of adult rats, *J Comp Neurol* **410**:42–54, 1999.

Cullheim S, Carlstedt T, Lindå H *et al.*, Motoneurons reinnervate skeletal muscle after ventral root implantation into the spinal cord of the cat, *Neuroscience* **29**:725–733, 1989.

Cullheim S, Carlstedt T, Risling M, Axon regeneration of spinal cord motoneurons following a lesion at the cord–ventral root interface. From basic animal research to a new surgical approach in human cases of ventral root avulsion lesions. A review, *Spinal Cord* **37**:811–819, 1999.

Fraher JP, The maturation of the ventral root–spinal cord transitional zone. An ultrastructural study, *J Neurol Sci* **36**:427–449, 1978.

Fraher JP, The CNS–PNS transitional zone of the rat. Morphometric studies at cranial and spinal levels, *Progr Neurobiol* **38**:261–316, 1992.

Fransson P, Quantitative electron-microscopic observations on the non-neuronal cells and lipid droplets in the posterior funiculus of the cat after dorsal rhizotomy, *J Comp Neurol* **231**:490–499, 1985.

Frisen J, Haegerstrand A, Fried K *et al.*, Adhesive/repulsive properties in the injured spinal cord: relation to myelin phagocytosis by invading macrophages, *Exp Neurol* **129**:183–193, 1994.

Frisen J, Haegerstrand A, Risling M *et al.*, Spinal axons in central nervous system scar tissue are closely related to laminin-immunoreactive astrocytes, *Neuroscience* **65**:293–304, 1995.

Frisen J, Verge VM, Cullheim S *et al.*, Increased levels of trkB mRNA and trkB protein-like immunoreactivity in the injured rat and cat spinal cord, *Proc Natl Acad Sci U S A* **89**:11282–11286, 1992,

Frisen J, Verge VM, Fried K *et al.*, Characterisation of glial trkB receptors: different response to injury in the central and peripheral nervous system, *Proc Natl Acad Sci U S A* **90**:4971–4975, 1993.

Gordon T, Sulaiman O, Boyd JG, Experimental strategies to promote functional recovery after peripheral nerve injuries, *J Peripher Nerv Syst* **8**:236–250, 2003.

Hallin R, Carlstedt T, Nilsson-Remahl IA, Risling M, Spinal cord implantation of avulsed ventral roots in primates: correlation between restored motor function and morphology, *Exp Brain Res* **124**:304–310, 1999.

Hammarberg H, Risling M, Hokfelt T *et al.*, Expression of insulin-like growth factors and corresponding binding proteins (IGFBP-6) in rat spinal cord and peripheral nerve after axonal injuries, *J Comp Neurol* **400**:57–72, 1998.

Havtorn L, Kellerth JO, Regeneration by supernumerary axons with synaptic terminals in spinal motoneurons in cats, *Nature* **325**:711–714, 1987.

Hoffman CFE, Marani E, Oestreicher AB, Tomeer RTWM, Ventral root avulsion of the cat spinal cord at the brachial plexus level (cervical 7), *Eur J Morphol* **28**:418–429, 1990.

Horvat JC, Pecot-Dechavassine M, Mira JC, Reinnervation fonctionnelle d'un muscle squelettique du rat adulte au moyen d'un greffon de nerf périphérique introduit dans la moelle épinière par voie dorsale, *Comptes Rend Acad Sci III* **304**:143–148, 1987.

Hu P, McLachlan EM, Selective reactions of cutaneous and muscle afferent neurons to peripheral nerve transaction in rats, *J Neurosci* **19**:10559–10567, 2003.

Johansson CB, Momma S, Clarke DL, Identification of neuronal stem cell in the adult mammalian central nervous system, *Cell* **96**:25–34, 1999.

Kaas JH, Plasticity of sensory and motor maps in adult mammals, *Annu Rev Neurosci* **14**:137–167, 1991.

Kliot M, Smith GM, Siegal JD, Silver J, Astrocyte-polymer implants promote regeneration of dorsal root fibres into the adult mammalian spinal cord, *Exp Neurol* **109**:57–69, 1990.

Koliatsos VE, Price WL, Pardo CA, Price DL, Ventral root avulsion: an experimental model of death of adult motor neurons, *J Comp Neurol* **342**:35–44, 1994.

Korsching S, The neurotrophic factor concept: a reexamination, *J Neurosci* **13**:2739–2751, 1993.

Li Y, Carlstedt T, Berthold CH, Raisman G, Interaction of transplanted olfactory-ensheathing cells and host astrocytic processes provides a bridge for axons to regenerate across the dorsal root entry zone, *Exp Neurol* **188**:300–308, 2004.

Li Y, Field PM, Raisman G, Repair of adult rat corticospinal tract by transplants of olfactory ensheathing cells, *Science* **277**:2000–2002, 1997.

Li L, Wu W, Lin F *et al.*, Rescue of adult mouse motoneurons from injury-induced cell death by glial cell line–derived neurotrophic factor, *Proc Natl Acad Sci U S A* **92**:9771–9775, 1995.

Lindå H, Cullheim S, Risling M, A light and electron microscopic study of intracellularly HRP-labeled lumbar motoneurons after intramedullary axotomy in the adult cat, *J Comp Neurol* **318**:188–208, 1992.

Lindå H, Risling M, Cullheim S, "Dendraxons" in regenerating motoneurons in the cat: do dendrites generate new axons after central axotomy? *Brain Res* **358**:329–333, 1985.

Lindå H, Risling M, Shupliakov O, Cullheim S, Changes in the synaptic input to lumbar motoneurons after intramedullary axotomy in the adult cat, PhD thesis, Karolinska Institutet, Stockholm, Sweden, 1993.

Lindholm T, Skold MK, Suneson A *et al.*, Semaphorin and neuropilin expression in motoneurons after intraspinal motoneuron axotomy, *Neuroreport* **15**:649–654, 2004.

Livesey FJ, Fraher JP, Experimental traction injury of the cervical spinal nerve roots: a scanning EM study of rupture pattern in fresh tissue, *Neuropathol Appl Neurobiol* **18**:376–386, 1992.

MacKinnon S, Dellon L, O'Brian J, Changes in nerve fibre numbers distal to a nerve repair in the rat sciatic nerve model, *Muscle Nerve* **14**:1116–1122, 1991.

Mannion RJ, Woolf CJ, Pain mechanisms and management: a central perspective, *Clin J Pain* **16**:144–156, 2000.

Murray M, Goldberger M, Replacement of synaptic terminals in lamina II and Clarks' nucleus after unilateral lumbosacral dorsal rhizotomy in adult cats, *J Neurosci* **6**:3205–3217, 1986.

Nomura H, Furuta A, Iwaki T, Dorsal root rupture injury induces extension of astrocytic processes into the peripheral nervous system and expression of GDNF in astrocytes, *Brain Res* **950**:21–30, 2002.

Novikov L, Novikova L, Kellerth JO, Brain-derived neurotrophic factor promotes axonal regeneration and long-term survival of adult rat spinal motoneurons *in vivo*, *Neuroscience* **79**:765–774, 1997.

Olsson T, Lundberg C, Lidman O, Piehl F, Genetic regulation of nerve avulsion-induced spinal cord inflammation, *Ann N Y Acad Sci* **917**:186–196, 2000.

Oorschot DE, Jones DG, Axonal regeneration in the mammalian central nervous system: a critique of hypotheses, *Adv Anat Embryol Cell Biol* **199**:1–121, 1990.

Oosthuyse B, Moons L, Storkebaum E *et al.*, Deletion of the hypoxia-response element in the vascular endothelial growth factor promoter causes motor neuron degeneration, *Nat Genet* **28**:131–138, 2001.

Ovelmen-Levitt J, Abnormal physiology of the dorsal horn as related to the deafferentation syndrome, *Appl Neurophysiol* **51**:104–116, 1988.

Pasterkamp RJ, Giger RJ, Verhagen J, Regulation of semaphorin III/collapsin-1 gene expression during peripheral nerve regeneration, *Exp Neurol* **153**:313–327, 1998.

Piehl F, Hammarberg H, Tabar G *et al.*, Changes in the MRNA expression pattern, with special reference to calcitonin gene-related peptide, after axonal injuries in rat motoneurons depends on age and type of injury, *Exp Brain Res* **119**:191–204, 1998.

Ramer MS, Priestley JV, McMahon SB, Functional regeneration of sensory axons into the adult spinal cord, *Nature* **403**:312–316, 2000.

Ramon-Cueto A, Nieto-Sampedro M, Regeneration into the spinal cord of transected dorsal root axons is promoted by ensheathing glial transplants, *Exp Neurol* **127**:232–244, 1994.

Reier PJ, Stensaas LJ, Guth L, The astrocytic scar as an impediment to regeneration in the central nervous system, in Kao CC (ed.), *Spinal Cord Reconstruction*, Raven Press, New York, pp. 163–195, 1983.

Risling M, Cullheim S, Hildebrand C, Reinnervation of the ventral root L7 from ventral horn neurons following intramedullary axotomy in adult cats, *Brain Res* **280**:15–23, 1983.

Risling M, Fried K, Lindå H *et al.*, Regrowth of motor axons following spinal cord lesions: distribution of laminin and collagen in the CNS scar tissue, *Brain Res Bull* **30**:405–414, 1993.

Saldanha G, Bar KJ, Yiangou Y *et al.*, Marked increase of interleukin-6 in injured human nerves and dorsal root ganglia, *J Neurol Neurosurg Psychiatr* **69**:692–709, 2000.

Schwab ME, Caroni P, Oligodendrocytes and CNS myelin are nonpermissive substances for neurite growth and fibroblast spreading *in vitro*, *J Neurosci* **8**:2381–2393, 1988.

Sims TJ, Gilmore SA, Interactions between intraspinal Schwann cells and the cellular constituents normally occurring in the spinal cord: an ultrastructural study in the irradiated rat, *Brain Res* **276**:17–30, 1983.

Sindou M, Quoex C, Baleydier C, Fibre organisation at the posterior spinal cord–rootlet junction in man, *J Comp Neurol* **153**:15–26, 1974.

Sköld MK, Marti HH, Lindholm T *et al.*, Induction of HIF-1α but not HIF-2α in motoneurons after ventral funiculus axotomy — implication in neuronal survival strategies, *Exp Neurol* **188**:20–32, 2004.

Smith KJ, Kodama RT, Reinnervation of denervated skeletal muscle by central neurons regenerating via ventral roots implanted into the spinal cord, *Brain Res* **551**:221–229, 1991.

Soker S, Takasima S, Miao HQ *et al.*, Neuropilin-1 is expressed by endothelial and tumor cells as an isoform-specific receptor for vascular endothelial growth factor, *Cell* **92**:735–745, 1998.

Wictorin K, Björklund A, Axon outgrowth from grafts of human embryonic spinal cord in the lesioned adult rat spinal cord, *Neuroreport* **3**:1045–1048, 1992.

Zhao S, Pang Y, Beuerman R *et al.*, Expression of c-Fos protein in the spinal cord after brachial plexus injury: comparison of root avulsion and distal nerve transection, *Neurosurgery* **42**:1357–1362, 1998.

7

SURGICAL EXPOSURES AND REPAIRS

Brachial and lumbosacral plexus lesions call for urgent surgical treatment. Indication for surgery is a violent trauma, often from road traffic accidents, resulting in complete or partial loss of function in the affected limb. Integrity of the spinal column must be ascertained preoperatively, by means of MRI or CT scans. An impact to the upper part of the body with thoracoscapular dissociation quite often also means a trauma to the head and neck with a potential instability in the cervical spine. With regards to the lower limbs, fractures of the spine, pelvis, or femur come almost always together with a lumbosacral plexus injury.

Head or chest injuries have priority, but treatment of the nerve injury is imperative. Surgery should be performed as soon as possible in order to obtain the best functional outcome, as the success of regeneration is determined to a large extent by processes that occur immediately following the injury (Fu and Gordon 1997). A delay in nerve regeneration conspires together with atrophy and degeneration of denervated organs to increase the risk of permanent disability. Therefore, a wait-and-see attitude after such an injury, when soft tissue damage can be suspected, is not up to the standards of modern scientific nerve surgery.

Exposures

Brachial plexus

Extraspinal exposure. For a routine exposure of the supraclavicular brachial plexus, the patient is in a supine beach-chair position. After injection of local anaesthetic with adrenalin for haemostasis, a transverse skin incision almost parallel to the clavicle and some 2–3 cm above it is performed (Figs. 4 and 7). This is the preferred approach, as it gives full and easy access to the brachial plexus and the scar is cosmetically acceptable. Care should be taken to preserve the supraclavicular nerves, for sensation in this region and also for use in the reconstruction of the plexus lesion, when they can be applied as transfers. Skin flaps with subcutaneous fat and platysma are raised. A nice plane of dissection to raise the flaps is deep into the platysma. The external jugular vein should be spared; but sometimes, due to a variable and disturbing course, it has to be divided. Next, dissection is made in the fat pad near the jugular vein or the lateral part of the sternocleidomastoid muscle, which sometimes can be quite wide at its insertion into the clavicle. Therefore, the most lateral part of the muscle sometimes needs to be detached in order to dissect toward the brachial plexus. It is now quite easy to feel the ridge formed by the sometimes scarred plexus. The omohyoid muscle, which is a key point in this dissection, is reached in this lower medial part of the posterior triangle. The muscle consists of two bellies separated by an intermediate tendon. Deeper in the fat pad are the superficial transverse cervical vessels, which are tied. By then, the anterior scalene muscle should be seen, as well as the phrenic nerve. This leads in cranial direction to the proximal C5 spinal nerve. In cases of complete proximal rupture, a stump of C5 is often concealed, but can be retrieved deep near the phrenic nerve and into the mouth of the C5 foramen. The most proximal parts of the other nerves of the plexus, e.g. C6–T1, are found deep near to the lateral part of the scalenus anterior. This muscle can be resected in order to display the proximal parts of the nerves, protecting the phrenic nerve. The lower trunk, C8 and T1, is situated behind the subclavian artery. The deep transverse cervical vessels usually leave the subclavian artery there, and project laterally in between the C8 and C7 nerves. As this artery is sometimes embedded in scar tissue, an irritating bleeding can evolve if care is not taken.

When there has been a severe traction injury and the origin of the brachial plexus has ruptured, it is usually displaced to underneath the clavicle. In order to mobilise the retroclavicular or infraclavicular brachial plexus, it is sometimes necessary, particularly if there has been a delay between trauma and operation and there is scarring, to extend the incision into the deltopectoral groove and cut the clavicle. On the other hand, when surgery is done early after the accident, the displaced plexus can be easily retrieved, even if it is underneath the clavicle (see also Birch *et al.* 1998).

Endoscopy. When there are avulsions and the spinal nerve and roots have been pulled out of the spinal and intervertebral canal, it is possible to introduce an endoscope through the empty foramen. The first endoscopic study to assess structures of the spinal canal were done in cadavers (Burman 1931), followed by the development of a myeloscope which was used for inspection of the cauda equina by way of a standard lumbar puncture (Pool 1942). With modern techniques, the myeloscopes have become more and more refined.

Today, this instrument is mainly used for decompression of nerve roots and disc surgery, but can be introduced through the intervertebral foramina (Ditsworth 1998). A percutaneous technique to visualise the intraspinal part of the brachial plexus, but not through the foraminal approach, has been described (Monsivais *et al.* 1994). At present, in severe brachial plexus injuries, a small 2 mm in diameter joint arthroscope is used. The lower foramina, i.e. the C7–T1 intervertebral canal, is best suited for this manoeuvre as it is larger than the foramina above and does not contain the vertebral vessels. More information regarding remaining intradural root stumps or full root avulsions can be gained with this technique than through ancillary investigations (e.g. electrophysiology or CT myelography), particularly regarding the lower roots of the brachial plexus without proceeding to full inspection after a laminectomy (Fig. 1).

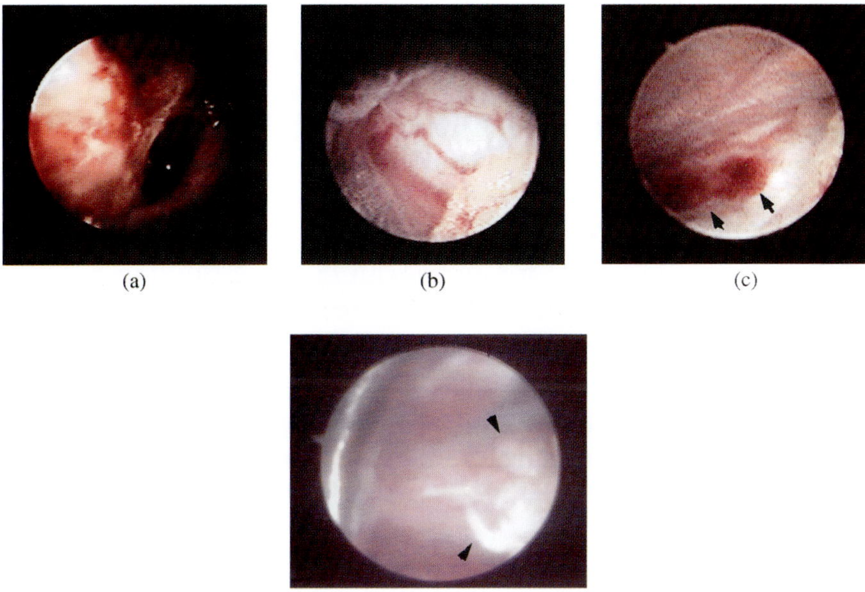

Fig. 1 Endoscopy of cervical spinal cord through empty intervertebral foramina after brachial plexus avulsion injury. (a) At the foramen. (b) Spinal cord with vessels in pia mater is seen through the endoscope. (c) Small bleedings at the site of root avulsion (arrows). (d) Root stump in the spinal canal (arrowheads).

Case 1. An 18-year-old man involved in a road traffic accident sustained a posterior fossa subdural haematoma, a compound fracture of his right femur, a right lung effusion, and a right brachial plexus injury. He had a complete flail right upper extremity with no activity in the serratus anterior. There was an ipsilateral Horner sign, but no Tinel's sign, when tapping over the site of the brachial plexus in the posterior triangle of the neck. Clinically, he seemed to have sustained a complete avulsion of the right brachial plexus; but a CT myelogram indicated roots from C5, C6, and possibly C7. Some tufts from C8 and T1 were apparent. At surgery, stumps were found in the foramina of C5 and C6 and were used for reconstruction. A small joint endoscope was introduced into the foramina of C7, C8, and T1. A good stump was found in the canal of C8 [Fig. 1(d)], but nothing in the intervertebral canal of C7 and T1. The ruptured ventral roots at C7, C8, and T1 were fed into the canal of C8 with fine forceps under endoscopic control to appose the stump in the canal. Their position was retained by Tisseal glue. Nerve grafts were based on the intraforaminal stumps of C5 and C6. There was a slow recovery of function in the shoulder as well as elbow flexion and extension.

Exposure of the most proximal part of the brachial plexus, medial to the external vertebral foramina, can be done through a dorsal approach (Kline *et al.* 1978; Smith *et al.* 1986; Kline *et al.* 1992; Carlstedt *et al.* 1995), an anterior approach (George *et al.* 1999; Fournier *et al.* 2001), or a lateral exposure (Kratimenos and Crockard 1993). In cases of most proximal ruptures of the spinal nerve within the intervertebral canal, an intraforaminal exposure is a safe and good approach together with the subscapular dissection of the supraclavicular brachial plexus (Kline *et al.* 1978; Birch *et al.* 1998). The patient is positioned prone. A long curved paramedian skin incision from the upper cervical region to about T8 or to the lower part of the scapula is done. All of the trapezius and rhomboid muscles are detached through their tendons at the spine. The thin serratus posterior superior muscle is also detached medially. This is medial to the accessory nerve and the dorsal scapular nerve, which are protected by this incision. The shoulder blade can be freed from the thoracic wall by placing a hand underneath and pushing laterally, and retained in this position with a deep retractor. When doing so, the terminal parts of the transversa colli are seen and can be divided. It is now possible to reach the posterior triangle of the neck and the brachial plexus after the first rib has been defined (see Kline *et al.* 1978; Fournier *et al.* 2001). The second rib is more prominent; in order to reach the most medial parts of the first rib, the intercostalis externus muscle as well as the longissimus and splenius capitis muscles are here divided. The insertion of the posterior and the middle scaleni muscles are detached from the rib, after which the posterior part of the first rib can be removed if necessary. This is also an excellent route to tumours of the lower spinal nerves of the brachial plexus, which can occupy the upper thoracic aperture and displace the apex of the lung. For an approach to the intraforaminal part of the brachial plexus, the paraspinal muscles on the operating side are dissected free from the laminae, and then the spinous and articular processes are retracted to reach the facet joints and the lateral part of the laminae. This is occasionally time-consuming, as the origin of these muscles is complex and there are numerous venous plexuses in this region. After a lateral laminectomy, the intervertebral canal is opened from medial to lateral (see Kline *et al.* 1992).

Case 2. A young woman was involved in a road traffic accident and sustained a multitrauma. At the collision, she was hit at the base of her neck by timber sticking out from the back of a lorry. There was a right-sided hemopneumothorax, a crush fracture of the first right rib, fractures of the right transverse processes of the C7 and T1 vertebrae, and lesions in her right brachial plexus. There was weakness in shoulder and elbow function, and complete loss of function in hand muscles. There was no sensation in the ulnar part of the hand and forearm, with reduced sensation in the third finger but normal sensation in the two radial fingers. There was a Horner sign. A preoperative diagnosis of a severe C7–T1 proximal brachial plexus lesion was made. The patient was operated on about 1 week after the accident. It was decided to use the dorsal subscapular approach to the brachial plexus because the pattern of neurological deficit was somewhat unusual, as was the trauma. From the history and the findings of fractures to the transverse processes of the C7 and T1 vertebrae, a most proximal (possibly intraspinal) lesion could be suspected.

At surgery, the spinal nerves C5–C7 were found in continuity to their foramina. The C8 and T1 nerves had been dislodged from the spine. Electrical stimulation and SSEP of C5 and C6 yielded good responses distally as well as centrally. The C7 was "silent" on stimulation. After a limited laminectomy and drilling opened the foramina of C8 and T1, stumps proximal to the dorsal root ganglia were found at both levels (Fig. 2). The proximal C8 and T1 stumps were reconnected to their spinal nerves by means of nerve grafts (Fig. 2). There was a slow recovery of wrist and finger extension, indicating an axonotmesis lesion for C7. About 1–1.5 years after the injury, there was return of muscle function in extrinsic

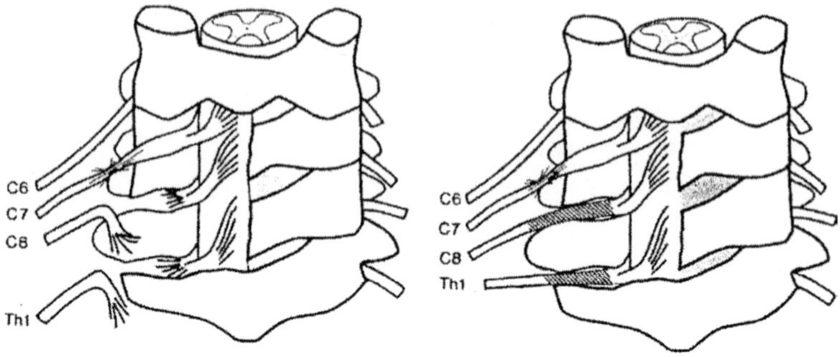

Fig. 2 Schematic drawings showing (left) brachial plexus injury and (right) repair with nerve grafts (hatched areas) (from Carlstedt and Noren 1995).

hand muscles innervated by the ulnar nerve; neither intrinsic muscle function nor sensation in the ulnar part of the hand recovered. In such a case, a conventional exposure of the brachial plexus would not have revealed the proximal stumps within or proximal to the vertebral foramina. Although there was not a full restitution of function, an accurate diagnosis and the reconstruction of the motor connections from C8 and T1 were possible (see Carlstedt and Noren 1995).

Intraspinal exposure. Theoretically, the most appealing way to reach the ventral part of the spinal cord would obviously be along the trajectory of the spinal nerves. With the patient in the commonly used supine semisitting position, the entire brachial plexus — supraclavicular as well as infraclavicular — is exposed and an anterolateral approach to the cervical spine can be performed (Fournier *et al.* 2001). The vertebral artery needs to be isolated and protected. A multilevel partial removal of the vertebral bodies is performed, and fusion for stability is not needed (George *et al.* 1999; Fournier *et al.* 2001). The disadvantage of this procedure is the risk of irritating bleeding from the vertebral artery, the prominent ventrolateral epidural venous complexes, and the quite deeply situated spinal cord once the vertebral bodies have been removed. Orientation and reaching to the sites of ventral root exit zones on the ventral surface of the spinal cord is, however, quite difficult (and, in fact, not necessary). There is — as has been demonstrated previously (Cullheim *et al.* 1989) — growth of new axons through the white matter of the spinal cord from the motoneuron pools of the ventral horn. In fact, choosing the most ventral site for implantation, where the ventral horn is near the surface of the spinal cord, involves a certain risk of compromising the motoneurons by the direct trauma of implantation. Of course, this approach is less favourable, if not impossible, if dorsal root reimplantation is intended.

The method of choice seems to be a lateral approach, including a limited facetectomy. This exposure makes it possible to reach as far ventral as the ventral midline spinal artery as well as the dorsal root entry zones, and to explore the supraclavicular and infraclavicular brachial plexus. The patient is in a strict lateral position (Crockard and Rogers 1996; Kratimenos and Crockard 1993). The head is supported in a Mayfield clamp with the neck slightly flexed towards the opposite side (Fig. 3). The head-up position of the operating table is used to prevent venous congestion, particularly of the epidural veins. During the procedure, the operating table's tilting facilities can be used when going from medial to lateral exposures of the plexus. A skin incision from the jugulum into the posterior triangle of the neck toward and passing the spinous process of the C5 vertebra is performed (Figs. 4 and 7). Platysma and skin flaps are raised and held either by stay sutures or a thyroid retractor. Dissections are made first in the posterior triangle of the neck of the injured extraspinal part of the brachial plexus and the accessory spinal nerve as it emerges from the posterior aspect of the sternocleidomastoid muscle (Fig. 5). The accessory nerve can be cut, as distal as possible, to be used later for transfer to the suprascapular nerve (see Chap. 5).

The second part of the dissection is to reach the cervical spine in the posterior part of the incision. No further skin incision is needed to perform this dissection (Figs. 4 and 5). The posterior tubercles of the transverse processes of C4 to C7 can be palpated, and are followed in the dissection through a connective tissue plane between the levator scapula and the posterior and medial scalene muscles (Fig. 4). The longissimus muscle deep to this plane must be split longitudinally to expose the posterior tubercles of the transverse processes and

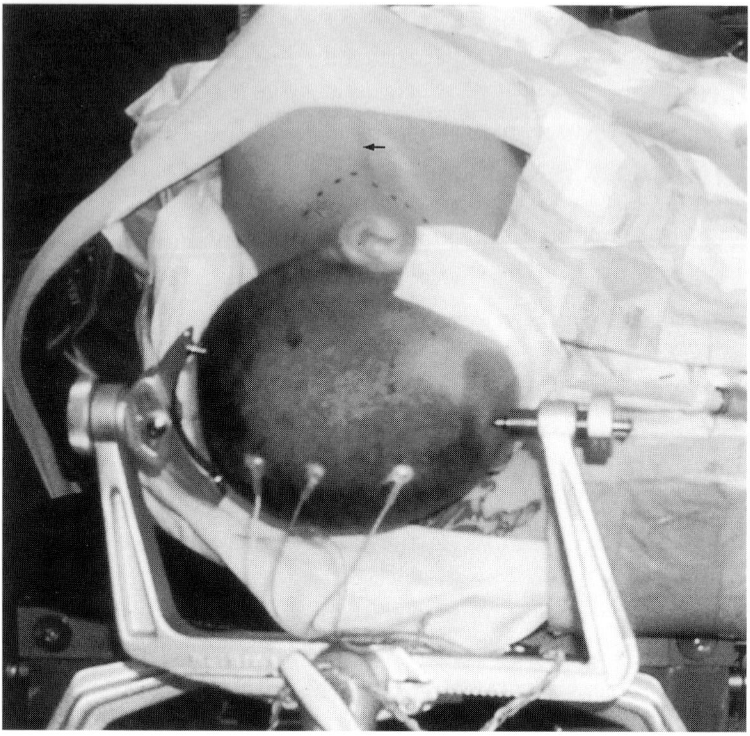

Fig. 3 Patient positioned laterally with head fixed in a Mayfield clamp and shoulder pulled down by Elastoplast. The skin incision is indicated. Note the ridge from the anterior part of the trapezius muscle (arrow). Electrodes for preoperative electrophysiological monitoring are applied to the scalp.

the hemilaminae (Fig. 4). The paravertebral muscles are detached from the hemilaminae and pushed dorsomedially. After a standard hemilaminectomy taking away the medial part of the processes at the facet joints using drills or rongeurs and breaching the periosteum (which could be confused with the dura mater), haemostasis of epidural veins, which laterally can cause irritating bleedings, is achieved. Sometimes, a rent in the dura mater is caused by the avulsion trauma and CSF starts to leak before the dura has been formally opened. The dura mater is incised longitudinally and stay sutures are applied (Fig. 6). The denticulate ligaments, usually preserved (Fig. 6), are cut from their lateral attachments. Stay sutures

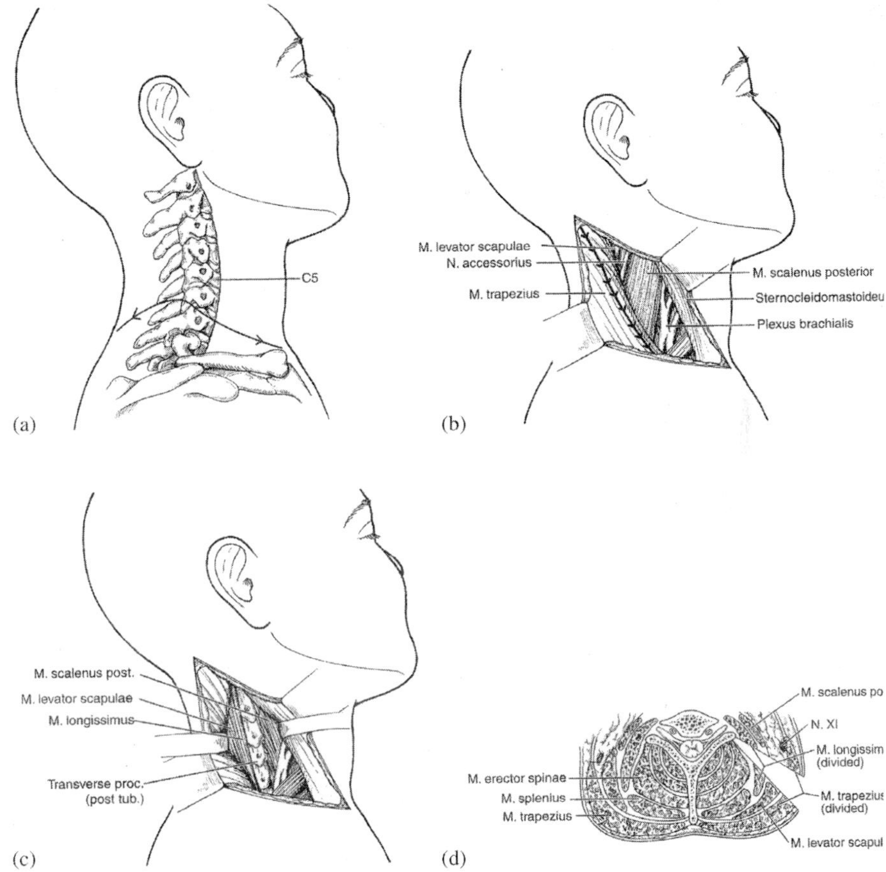

Fig. 4 Schematic drawings of the lateral approach to the brachial plexus. (a) A skin incision in the posterior triangle of the neck is extended toward the spinous process of C5 vertebra. (b) The trapezius muscle is divided according to the line with the arrows so that the accessory nerve is protected. [(c), (d)] Through a plane in between the levator scapulae and the scalenus muscles, the longissimus is reached and split longitudinally. The posterior tubercles of the transverse processes can now be seen (from Carlstedt and Birch 2000).

are applied to the part of the denticulate ligament that runs along the side of the spinal cord in order to gently rotate the cord (Fig. 6). With this approach, and with the help of the stay sutures in the denticulate ligament, it is possible to reach the anterior aspect of the spine at the ventral root exit zones. At this stage, it is possible to see

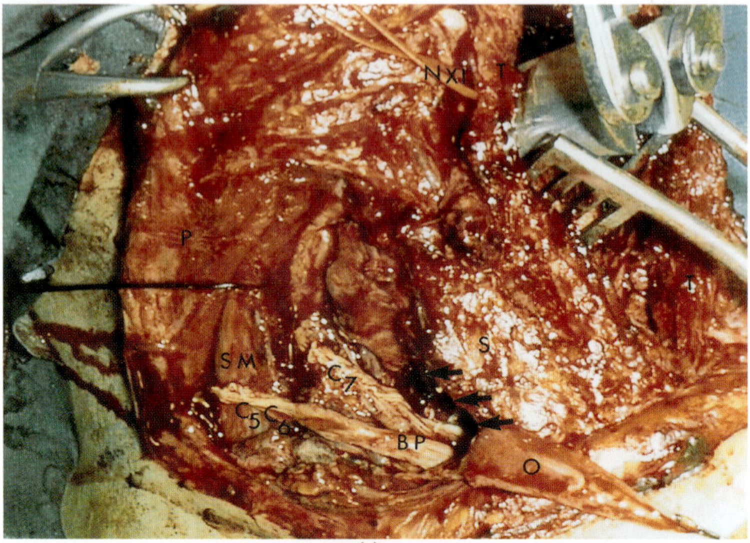

(a)

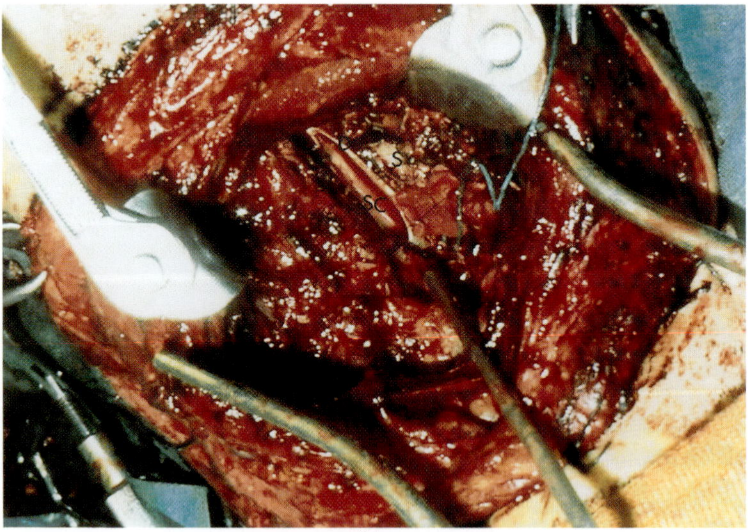

(b)

Fig. 5 Intraoperative pictures of exploration of (a) extraspinal and (b) intraspinal parts of brachial plexus. (a) The C5–C7 spinal nerves are avulsed from the spinal cord. Arrows indicate the empty foramina. There is a sling around the accessory nerve (NXI). A retractor is placed in the posterior part of the wound for the approach to the spine. (b) Lateral approach to the spine (S). The dura (D) has been opened and the spinal cord (SC) can be visualised (from Carlstedt *et al.* 2000).

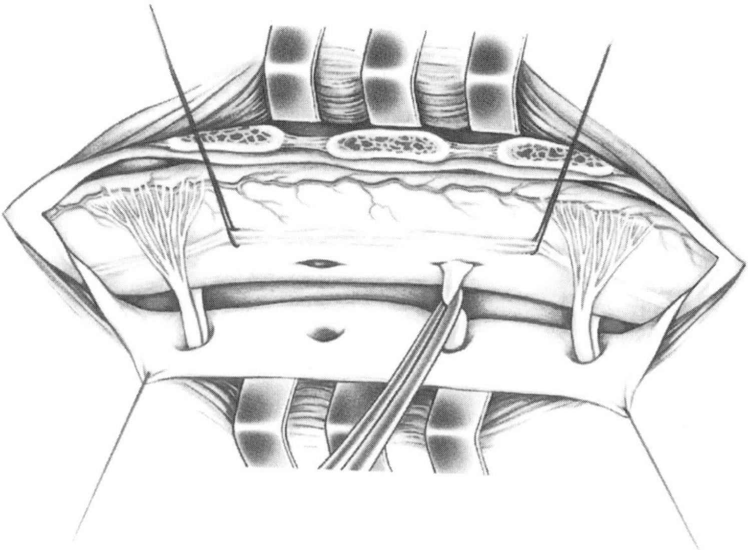

(a)

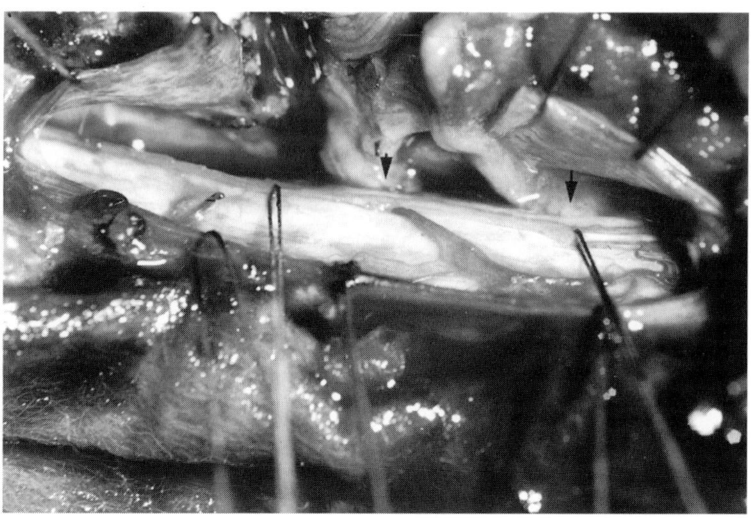

(b)

Fig. 6 Exposed spinal cord after the dura mater has been opened. Stay sutures are applied in the denticulate ligament. Through slits in the pia mater, a nerve graft has been implanted into the spinal cord. (a) Schematic drawing. (b) Intraoperative photograph (from Carlstedt *et al.* 2000).

if the roots have been completely avulsed and displaced outside the spinal canal (Fig. 7) or still remain within the subdural space in the spinal canal.

Case 3. (Fig. 7) A 9-year-old boy sustained a multitrauma when riding a motorcycle. There was a complete loss of function in the right upper extremity. A Tinel's sign could not be provoked, but there was a Horner sign. A preoperative CT myelogram showed signs of avulsions with meningoceles for the spinal nerves C5 to T1 (see Fig. 8, Chap. 4). Surgery was performed 4 weeks after the accident. The patient was positioned in a lateral position, his head secured in a Mayfield clamp, and a skin incision from the jugulum across the spinous process of C4 was made [Figs. 7(a) and 7(b)]. Simultaneous explorations of the extraspinal and intraspinal parts of the brachial plexus were done [Fig. 7(c)]. All spinal roots with dorsal root ganglia were found in the posterior triangle of the neck [Fig. 7(d)]. The right hemilaminae and articulate processes of the lower cervical spine were exposed [Fig. 7(e)]. A laminoplasty from C4 to C7 was done [Fig. 7(f)]. After the partially torn dura was opened, the finding from the CT myelogram of complete C5–T1 avulsion injury could be verified [Fig. 7(g)]. A silicon catheter introduced through the intervertebral canals served as a lead for the nerve grafts [Figs. 7(g) and 7(h)]. Reconstruction of the entire plexus through nerve grafts implanted into the spinal cord segment C5–C8 was performed (for outcome, see Chap. 8).

Lumbosacral plexus

The lumbar plexus is reached through a lateral retroperitoneal approach. The patient is in a lateral or semilateral position. The skin incision follows the iliac crest and curves proximally (see Fig. 3 in Chap. 5). The muscle origin is detached from the iliac crest. The peritoneum is defined and pushed medially to expose the lateral pelvic and abdominal wall. The approach can be extended distal to the iliac notch, where the lateral cutaneous nerve of the thigh enters the thigh, and more medially, detaching the inguinal ligament to

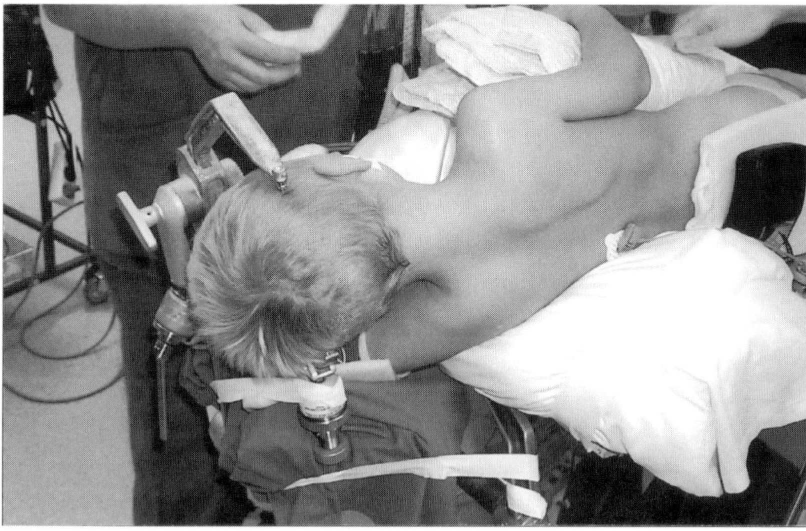

(a)

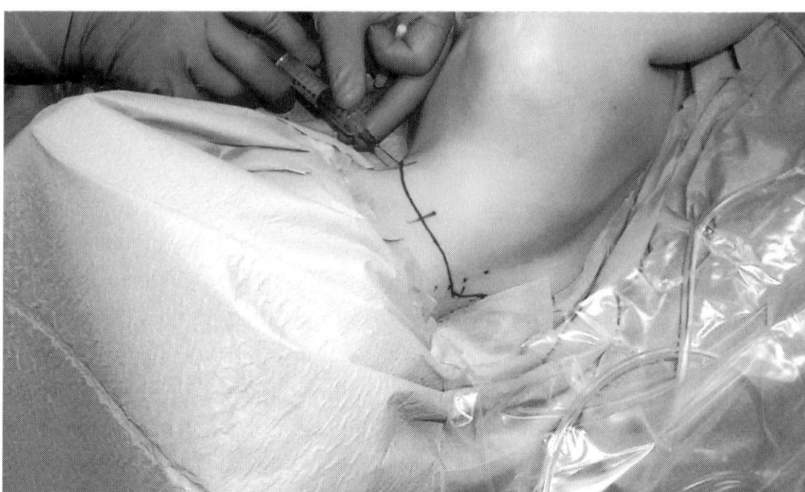

(b)

Fig. 7 A sequence of pictures taken through an operation for repair of a complete intraspinal brachial plexus avulsion injury. [(a), (b)] Position of patient. Indication and injection at site for skin incision. [(c), (d)] Simultaneous dissection in the posterior triangle of the neck and at the cervical spine. The avulsed brachial plexus is displayed in (d). [(e), (f)] The right side of the lower cervical spine with the lateral mass exposed. A laminoplasty is performed in (f). [(g), (h)] The partly torn dura opened. No remaining roots are found. A catheter is introduced through the C7 canal, with the other end in the posterior triangle of the neck ready to apply nerve grafts.

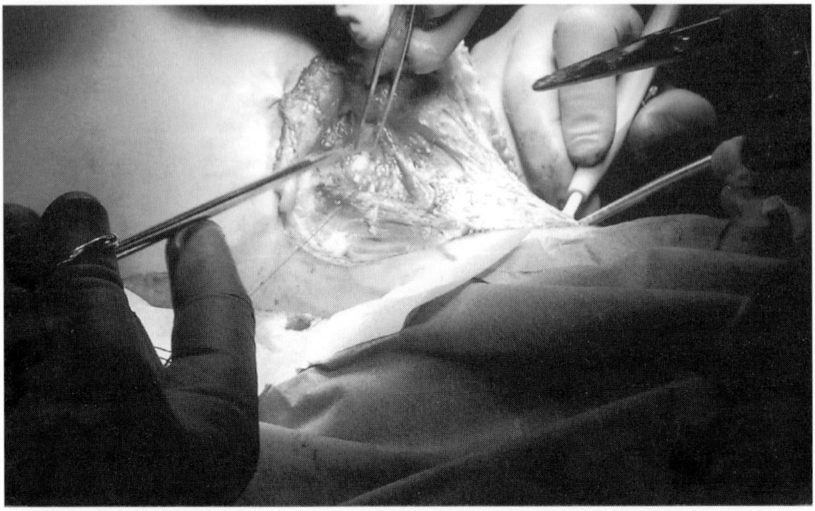

(c)

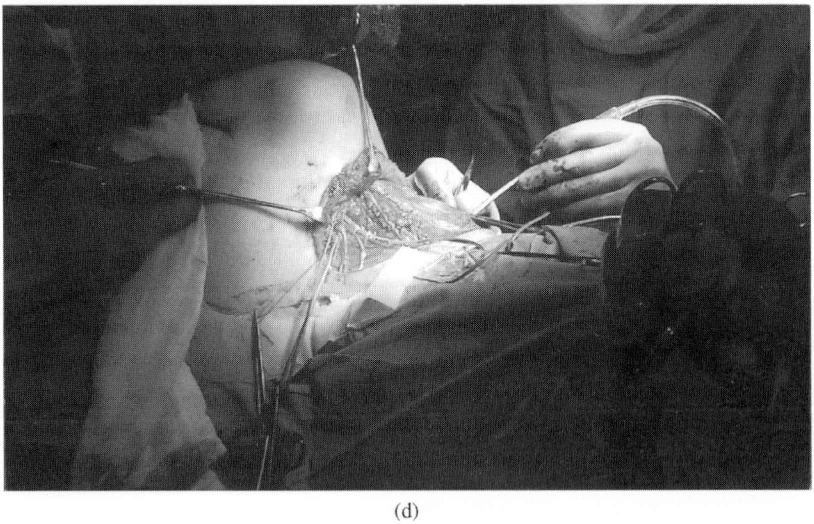

(d)

Fig. 7 (*Continued*)

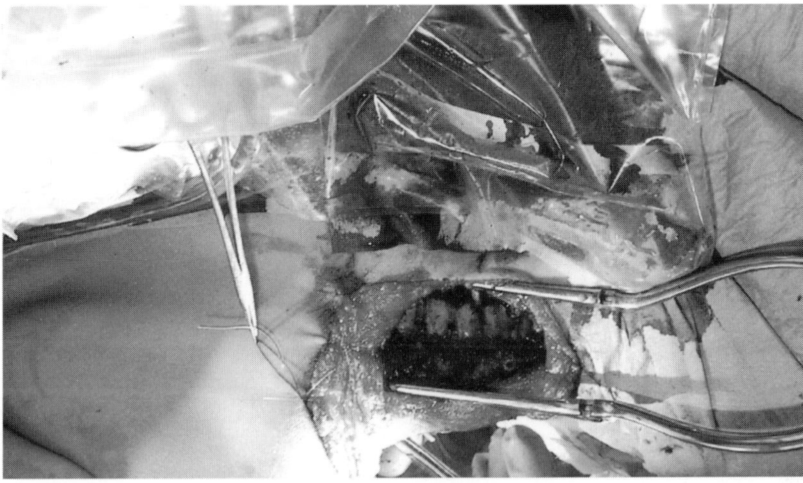

(e)

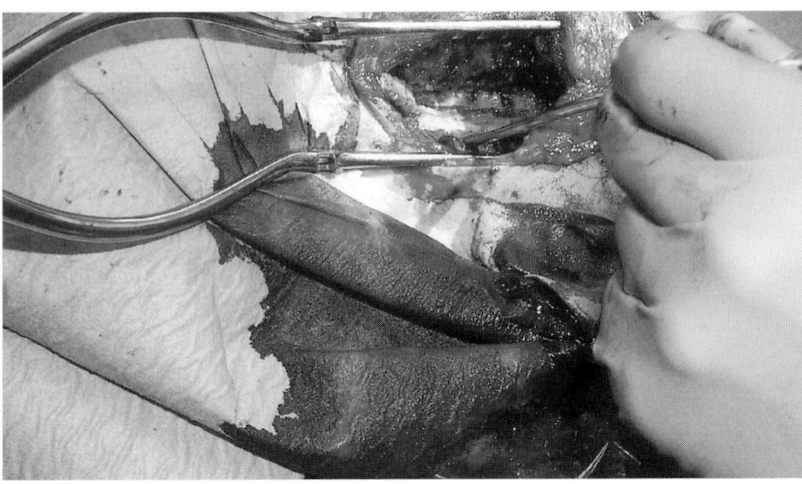

(f)

Fig. 7 (*Continued*)

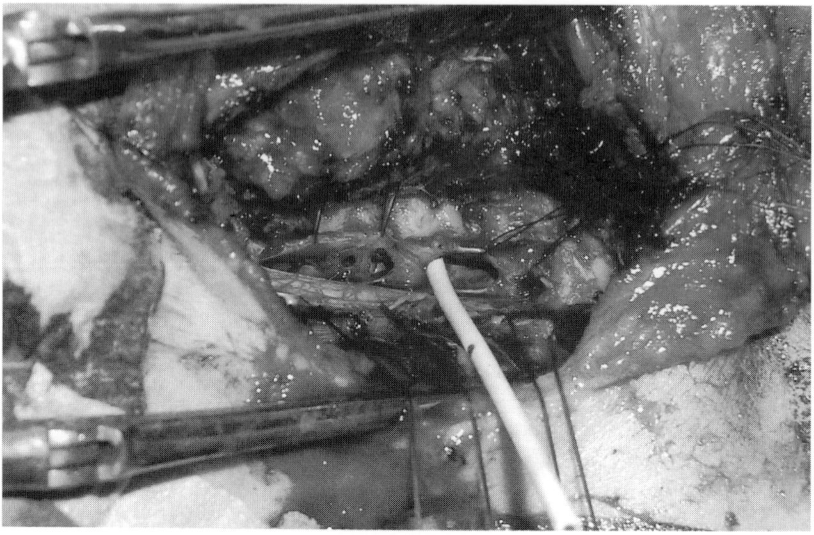

(g)

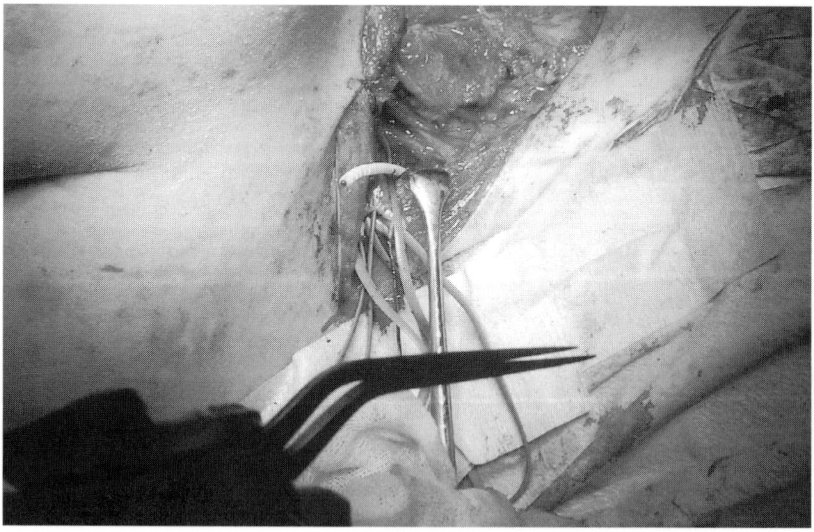

(h)

Fig. 7 (*Continued*)

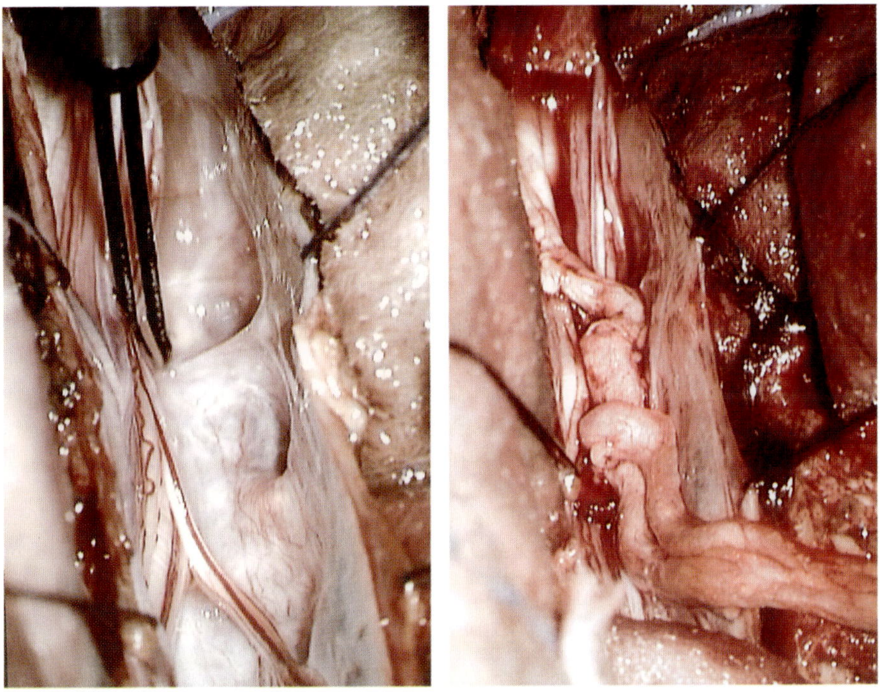

(a) (b)

Fig. 8 Intraoperative photographs of the sacral canal. (a) Empty foramina at L5, S1, and S2 *in situ*. (b) Sacral canal after sural nerve grafting to the proximal stump of the S1 ventral root (from Lang *et al.* 2004).

find the femoral nerve. In rostral and medial direction, the incision can extend to the lower ribs and the intercostal nerves. From the lateral border of psoas, the intrapelvic parts of the iliohypogastricus, the ilioinguinalis, and the lateral cutaneous nerve of the thigh are found; and more medially in the gutter between the iliacus and the psoas major muscles is the femoral nerve. Medial to the psoas muscles is the obturator nerve and, further to the midline deep near the great vessels, the lumbosacral trunk. The femoral nerve can be used as a guide to reach the lumbar plexus. The psoas muscles need to be detached or cut to expose the origin of the lumbar plexus.

The lumbar origin of the sacral plexus, i.e. the lumbosacral trunk, can be reached through this approach, but it is difficult to expose and manipulate the sacral plexus this way. A transperitoneal route through the lower abdomen is preferred (Kline and Hudson 1995). However, after an injury with the scarring around the sacral plexus and deep near the great vessels, this is also a very difficult dissection. Sedel (1975) has suggested a transiliac approach, after Judet, with a comfortable view of the whole lumbosacral plexus after osteotomy of the os ilium. The disadvantage of this operation is the disarticulation of the sacroiliac joint. Another possibility to explore the sacral plexus and the sciatic nerve at its point of exit at the sciatic notch is a dorsal transsacral approach, as has been described by Linarte and Gilbert (1986). This approach allows bypass grafts with a maximal length of 10–15 cm for L4 and L5, and about 5 cm for reconstruction at S3. This surgical technique is useful and has been only slightly modified.

For an approach to the distal parts of the sacral plexus and an intraspinal exploration of the sacral roots or the cauda equina, the patient is in prone position. A curved skin incision is made from the lower lumbar region along the iliac crest and caudally towards the tuber ischiadicum. The paraspinal muscles are detached from the L4 and L5 vertebrae and the sacrum. The spinous processes are removed, and the laminae as well as the dorsal sacrum to the dorsal lateral foramina are exposed. The foramina are opened to look for the dorsal rami and the sacral spinal nerves if *in situ*. It is now possible to extend the bone removal by performing a formal hemilaminectomy in the sacral spinal canal, as well as lower lumbar canal diagnosis and repair of spinal nerve or root ruptures after the dura has been opened (Fig. 8). The distal part of the torn and displaced sacral plexus is explored at the sciatic notch, after the medial origin of the gluteus maximus muscle has been detached. Through the same skin incision, the medial part of the gluteus maximus muscle is elevated from the sacrum and the posterior parts of the ilium. A dissection deep into the muscle follows. The piriform muscle is cut after the glutei nerves and vessels have been identified and protected. The glutei veins, if cut, could retract into the pelvis and cause severe haemorrhage. The gluteus superior nerve is of particular interest for the reconstruction to follow.

Findings from explorations of lumbosacral plexus injuries were that most cases of neurotmesis occurred as intraspinal or cauda equina injuries. In cases of fractures through the sacral foramina, the spinal nerves and roots appeared compressed or cut by the fracture. Root ruptures occurred between the spinal ganglion and the lumbar enlargement of the spinal cord, but there was no avulsion of the roots from the spinal cord. The distal root stumps with ganglia were sometimes pulled out of the spinal canal into the pelvis in front of the sacrum, and were therefore difficult to explore properly, particularly if there had been development of scar tissue. Occasionally, it was possible to retrieve the displaced roots and ganglia at the sciatic notch and perform an extra pelvic anastomosis by means of a nerve graft to the proximal ruptured ventral roots.

Repairs

Brachial plexus (see video)

The pia mater and the pia–glial membrane are carefully opened by means of a scalpel blade or fine scissors to create a 1–2-mm deep and wide opening (Fig. 6) (Carlstedt *et al.* 2000; Carlstedt *et al.* 2004). Detached nerve roots can be retrieved through the intervertebral foramen, if the surgery is performed within days after the accident. This is done with great care using a tube or a catheter, avoiding injury to the vertebral vessels. This is not possible if the surgery is delayed more than 2 weeks, as the displaced roots will be scarred and the intervertebral foramen sealed by scar tissue. In some cases, the avulsed roots can be situated within the subdural space, allowing for direct reimplantation. In most cases, however, nerve grafting is the only possibility to reconnect the spinal cord to the avulsed roots.

The nerve graft (taken preferentially from the superficial radial nerve, the medial cutaneous nerve of the ipsilateral forearm, or the sural nerve) is split into separate fascicles for two to four different spinal cord segments and introduced to a depth of about 1–2 mm by means of a probe, leaving another 2 mm of white matter to the ventral horn and the motoneuron pool (see video). A small Roton instrument in the shape of a hockey stick is useful in this manoeuvre; its "blade", being 1–2 mm in length, can be used as a depth gauge when implanting the root or the nerve graft. Implanted grafts are maintained in position by glue (Tisseal), or they can be stitched to the pia. The pia is slightly elastic and closes around the introduced tips of the nerve graft. In case of root ruptures, the nerve graft is directly apposed to the trimmed end of the ventral root stump. The nerve grafts are pulled through the intervertebral foramen for C7 or C8 spinal nerves (see video; Fig. 8). If the foramen is blocked, the grafts are passed through the incision in the dura and outside the vertebral canal. The grafts are connected to the avulsed roots in the posterior triangle of the neck, where they have been displaced by the traction trauma. During the intraspinal procedure, spinal cord monitoring of motor tract function (MEP), together with SEP, is performed.

Usually, the dura is not closed, but the opening in the dura is covered by artificial dura or a vein patch and Tisseal glue. A lumbar drain is applied for about 1 week to prevent the development of CFS leakage. The patient is mobilised after a week, but the arm is kept in a sling for a total of 6 weeks.

Lumbosacral plexus

Direct repair of ruptured sacral plexus in the pelvis can be done by means of nerve grafts [Fig. 9(a)] after a transabdominal and transperitoneal approach. Quite often, this is not possible, so bypassing the lesion with grafts from the sacral spinal nerves to the nerves for key functions in the leg has to be performed [Fig. 9(b)].

Case 4. A 20-year-old man had a complex pelvic fracture with dissociation of the sacroiliac joint and the lumbosacral plexus lesion L4–S2. The pelvis was stabilised with an external fixator. He was referred 10 months after the accident. There was no activity in the glutei muscles, hamstrings, or calf muscles, and weakness in the quadriceps and adductor muscles. There was no sensation on the posterior aspect of the thigh and below the knee. Electrophysiological assessment showed no activity in the peroneus and tibialis anterior

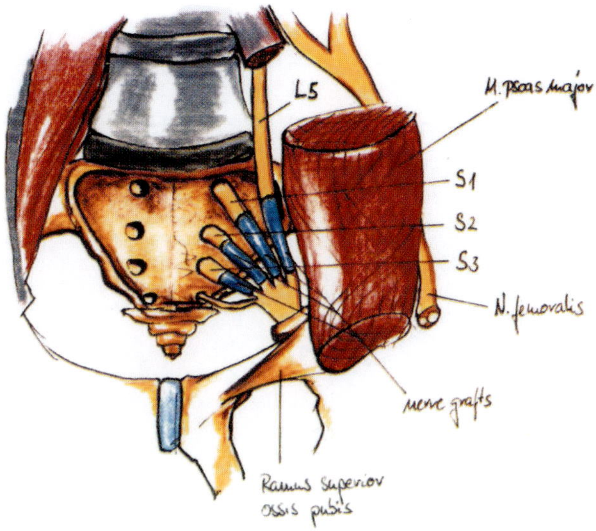

(a)

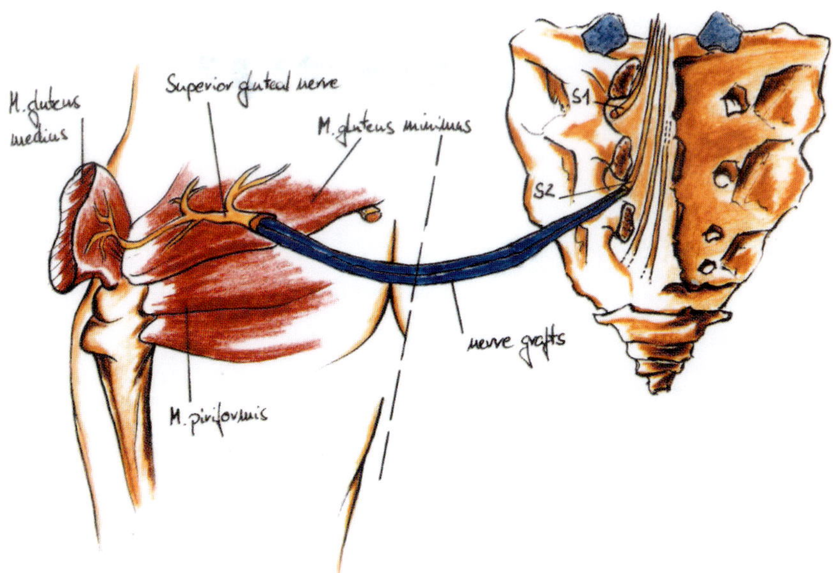

(b)

Fig. 9 Schematic repair strategies after sacral plexus lesions. (a) Intrapelvic repair with nerve grafts. (b) Intraspinal and extraspinal reconstruction of the sacral plexus for key functions by means of nerve grafts to gluteal and sciatic nerves. (c) Intraspinal repair of ruptured roots with nerve grafts (from Lang *et al.* 2004).

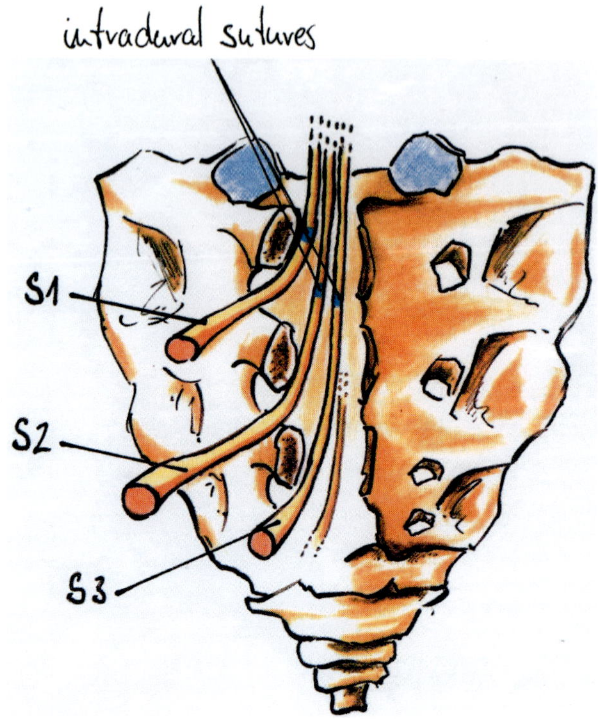

(c)

Fig. 9 (*Continued*)

muscles, and denervation activity with some motor units in the quadriceps. Through an anterior abdominal approach, a lesion of the lumbosacral plexus at L4–S3 was demonstrated. The proximal stumps at L5–S3 were connected by nerve grafts from the sural nerve to the distal intrapelvic part of the lumbosacral trunk.

Repair of the ventral roots, either directly or by means of interpositioned nerve grafts, can be performed early after injuries such as a transforaminal fracture of the sacrum. It is usually not possible to differentiate between proximal sensory and motor root stumps unless SEP is used, and therefore all proximal root stumps have to be involved in the repair.

Case 5. A 29-year-old man with a sacral fracture through the vertebral foramina had lost function distal to the knee. Electrophysiology demonstrated good activity in thigh muscles, but no volitional activity distal to the knee. Magnetic resonance imaging demonstrated cysts at S1–S3. A laminectomy was performed. It was possible to identify proximal and distal stumps for all three sacral roots. A repair by means of short sural nerve grafts was performed [Fig. 9(c)].

When the distal stumps of the lumbosacral plexus have slid through the foramina to the front of the sacroiliac area, they are difficult to retrieve (Kline *et al.* 1992). An intrapelvic exploration for distal stumps has poor chances of success and the risk is high. In such cases, it is therefore recommended to reconnect the intradural proximal stumps of the ventral roots with a sural nerve graft to a more distal part of the nerve or to the sciatic nerve outside the pelvis [Fig. 10(b)] (for surgical paradigms, see Fig. 12).

Case 6. A 3-year-old girl was hit by a car and sustained a trochanteric femoral fracture, fractures of the pelvis with sacroiliac joint dissociation, and ipsilateral fractures of the pubic rami with injuries to her internal organs, thus making a colostomy necessary. The pelvis was stabilised with an external fixator. Clinical assessment showed no activity in the territory of her right sacral plexus with loss of function in the glutei, hamstrings, and muscles below the knee. The result of the myelography was inconclusive with regard to an intradural lesion. A laminectomy from L5 to S2 was performed. The proximal root stumps of L5, S1, and S2 were found; however, the distal stumps were not found in the spinal canal. By dissection at the sciatic notch and by elevating the gluteus maximus muscle from its medial attachment, it was possible to retrieve the distal root stumps with ganglia. The three proximal nerve roots were reconnected by five strands of the sural nerve grafts to the sacral plexus outside the pelvis [Fig. 9(b)].

Case 7. A 22-year-old woman sustained a complicated pelvic fracture with sacroiliac joint dissociation in a road traffic accident. She

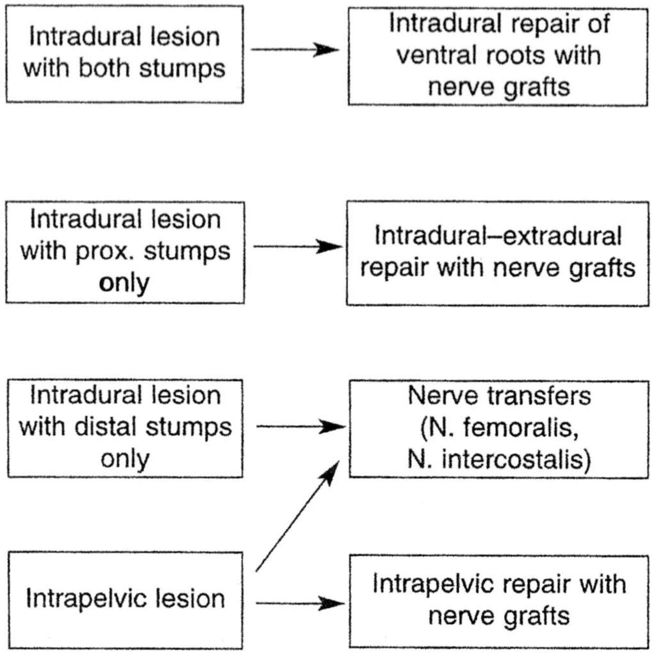

Fig. 10 Synopsis of surgical strategies for various lumbosacral plexus injuries. Prox.: proximal (from Lang *et al.* 2004).

had lost function in the left leg, except for femoral nerve function. On clinical examination, she had no activity in the hip extensors with a positive Trendelenburg's test. There was no hamstring or below-knee function. There was loss of sensation on the back of the thigh and in the sole of the foot. A CT myelogram showed intraspinal ruptures of L5, S1, and S2. It was possible to demonstrate proximal stumps on the scan. Based on that information, an intraspinal exploration of the sacral roots and cauda equina was performed. A laminectomy from L4 to S2 was performed. After the dura was opened, the proximal stumps of S1 and S2, but not L5, could be defined (Fig. 8). SEP demonstrated central connection of the sensory roots, and those that did not respond on SEP were used for reconstruction. The gluteal and sciatic nerves were dissected after the gluteus maximus muscle had been mobilised from its medial attachment. The S1 and S2 motor roots were connected through the nerve grafts to the gluteal and sciatic nerves [Figs. 8 and 9(b)].

Conclusion

The lateral position is preferred for an extraspinal and intraspinal approach to the brachial plexus. Spinal cord reimplantation is performed in the anterolateral aspect of the spinal cord through multiple small slits in the pia mater. The peripheral nerve graft or the avulsed root is introduced deep to the surface of the spinal cord. The lumbosacral plexus injury is approached according to the type of injury preperitoneally or retroperitoneally. In cases of ruptures of the cauda equina, the lumbosacral spinal canal is opened and root-to-nerve grafting is performed.

References

Birch R, Bonney G, Wynn Parry CB, *Surgical Disorders of the Peripheral Nerves*, Churchill Livingstone, Edinburgh, Scotland, 1998.

Burman MS, Myeloscopy or the direct visualisation of the spinal canal and its contents, *J Bone Joint Surg* **13**:695, 1931.

Carlstedt T, Anand P, Hallin R *et al.*, Spinal nerve root repair and reimplantation of avulsed ventral roots into the spinal cord after brachial plexus injury, *J Neurosurg* **93**:237–247, 2000.

Carlstedt T, Anand P, Htut M *et al.*, Restoration of hand function and so called "breathing arm" after intraspinal repair of C5–T1 brachial plexus avulsion injury. Case report, *Neurosurg Focus* **16**:article 7, 2004.

Carlstedt T, Birch R, Surgical management of nerve root injuries, in Schmidek HH (ed.), *Operative Neurosurgical Techniques*, 4th edn, Saunders, Philadelphia, PA, pp. 2369–2376, 2000.

Carlstedt T, Grane P, Hallin RG, Noren G, Return of function after spinal cord implantation of avulsed spinal nerve roots, *Lancet* **346**:1323–1325, 1995.

Carlstedt T, Noren G, Repair of ruptured spinal nerve roots in a brachial plexus lesion, *J Neurosurg* **82**:661–663, 1995.

Crockard HA, Rogers M, Open reduction of traumatic atlanto-axial rotatory dislocation with the use of the extreme lateral approach. A report of two cases, *J Bone Joint Surg [Am]* **78**:431–436, 1996.

Cullheim S, Carlstedt T, Lindå H *et al.*, Motoneurons reinnervate skeletal muscle after ventral root implantation into the spinal cord of the cat, *Neuroscience* **29**:725–733, 1989.

Ditsworth DA, Endoscopic transforaminal lumbar discetomy and reconfiguration: a posterolateral approach into the spinal canal, *Surg Neurol* **49**:588–597, 1998.

Fournier HD, Mercier P, Menei P, Anatomical bases of the posterior approach to the brachial plexus for repairing avulsed spinal nerve roots, *Surg Radiol Anat* **23**:3–38, 2001.

Fu SY, Gordon T, The cellular and molecular basis of peripheral nerve regeneration, *Mol Neurobiol* **14**:67–116, 1997.

George B, Gauthier N, Lot G, Multisegmental cervical spondylotic myelopathy and radiculopathy treated by multilevel oblique corpectomies without fusion, *Neurosurgery* **44**:81–90, 1999.

Kline DG, Donner TR, Happel L *et al.*, Intraforaminal repair of plexus spinal nerves by a posterior approach: an experimental study, *J Neurosurg* **76**:459–470, 1992.

Kline DG, Hudson AR, *Nerve injuries. Operative Results for Major Nerve Injuries, Entrapments, and Tumors*, WB Saunders, Philadelphia, PA, pp. 328–344, 1995.

Kline DG, Kott J, Barnes G, Bryant L, Exploration of selected brachial plexus lesions by the posterior subscapular approach, *J Neurosurg* **49**:872–880, 1978.

Kratimenos GP, Crockard HA, The far lateral approach for ventrally placed foramen magnum and upper cervical spine tumors, *Br J Neurosurg* **7**:129–140, 1993.

Lang EM, Borges J, Carlstedt T, Surgical treatment of lumbosacral plexus injuries, *J Neurosurg Spine* **1**:64–71, 2004.

Linarte R, Gilbert A, Trans-sacral approach to the sacral plexus, *Peripher Nerve Repair Regen* **4**:17–20, 1986.

Monsivais JJ, Narakas AO, Turkof E, Sun Y, The endoscopic diagnosis and possible treatment of nerve root avulsion in the management of brachial plexus injuries, *J Hand Surg [Br]* **19**:547–549, 1994.

Pool JL, Myeloscopy: intraspinal endoscopy, *Surgery* **11**:169–182, 1942.

Sedel L, Voies d'abord des nerfs du membre inférieur, *Med Chir Technol Chirurg Orthop (Paris)* **44530**:1–8, 1975.

Smith B, Hurst J, Richter H, Kline DG, Posterior laminotomy approach to brachial plexus roots in primates: graft repair evaluated by electromyography, *Surg Forum* **37**:487–489, 1986.

8

OUTCOME

Spinal nerve root injury from traction of the brachial or lumbosacral plexus is amenable to surgery with functional outcome. Among the unfavourable conditions that interfere with functional recovery are a delay in undergoing surgery, and the presence of associated severe injuries to the large vessels and the brain or the spinal cord.

Brachial Plexus

Motor recovery

Clinically, most patients were noted to recover muscle function within 1 year after the injury, witnessing muscle twitches (MRC grade 1/5), usually in the pectoral muscle (Carlstedt *et al.* 1995; Carlstedt *et al.* 2000; Htut *et al.* 2007). The first subclinical electrophysiological signs of muscle reinnervation occurred about 9–15 months after surgery. Muscle activity returned first in shoulder muscles, followed by upper arm muscles about a year later and, in a few cases, as far distally as to one or two forearm muscles during the third year (Fig. 1). There was an eventual increase in power in the shoulder girdle muscles — i.e. the serratus anterior, pectoral, and supraspinal muscles — to a significant power, in many cases reaching a normal magnitude of MRC 4–5/5. There was less power in the upper arm muscles, which never reached a normal (albeit still useful) level, i.e.

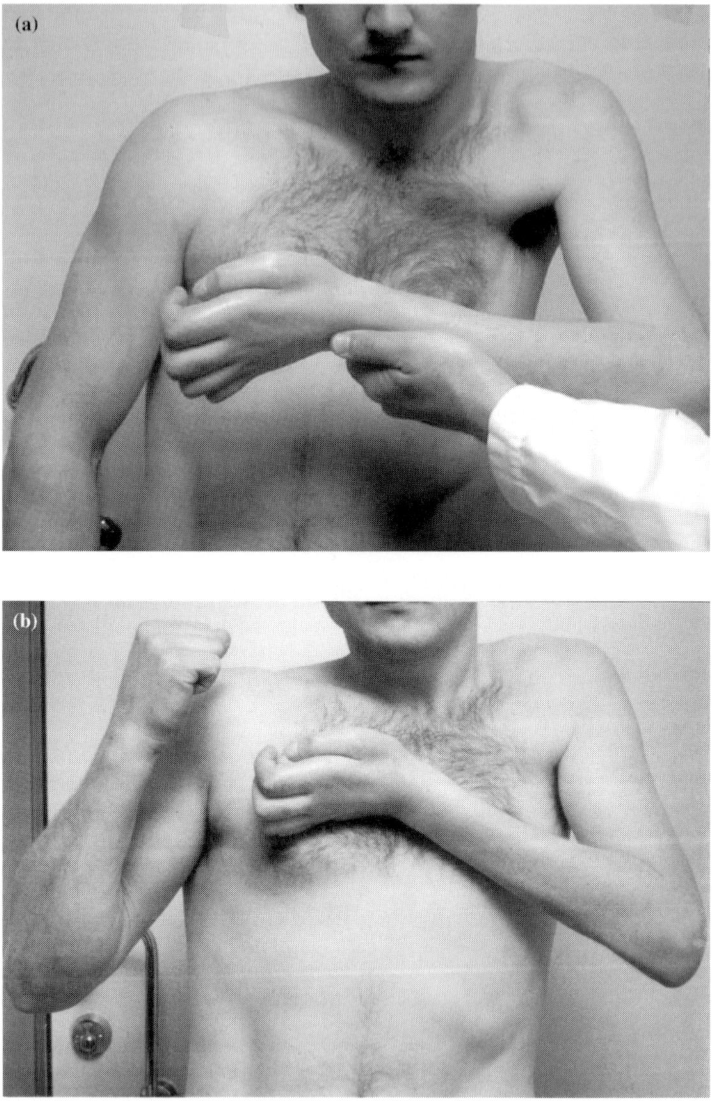

Fig. 1 Photographs showing the first operated human case of total brachial plexus injury 3 years after implantation of C6 ventral root directly into the pertinent spinal cord segment and reconnection of the avulsed C7 ventral root by means of nerve grafts implanted into the spinal cord. The avulsed C8 and T1 were not reconstructed. (a) Recovery of the clavicular part of the pectoral muscle. (b) The biceps muscle has regained 4/5 MRC power. The clavicular part of the pectoral muscle is cocontracting with elbow flexors. There is some activity (2/5) in the brachioradial muscle, but no hand function (Carlstedt *et al.* 2000). (c) After recovery, the patient could return to his previous work in a garage (Cullheim *et al.* 1999).

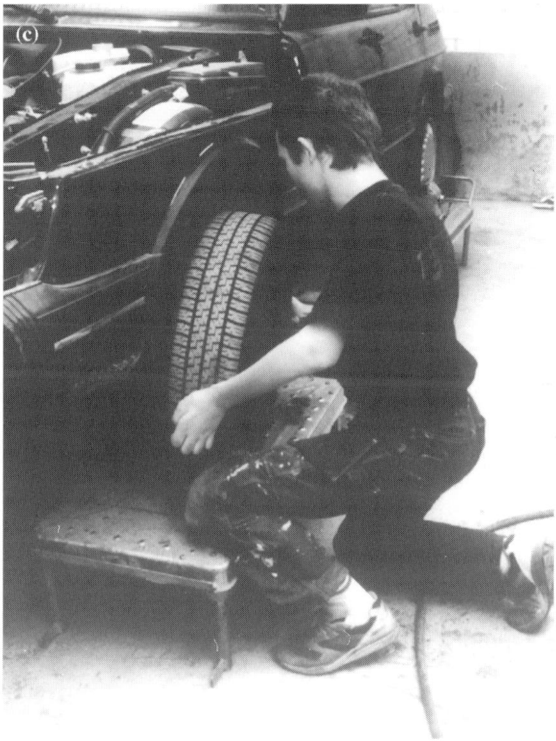

Fig. 1 (*Continued*)

MRC 3–4/5 (Fig. 1). Muscle power in the brachioradial and flexor carpi radial muscles reached only about MRC 2/5, i.e. they were not functionally useful (Carlstedt *et al.* 1995; Carlstedt *et al.* 2000). Obviously, this is not a case of specific motoneuron-to-original-target regeneration. The regrowing new axons try to reinnervate the first possible muscle target, i.e. the shoulder muscles. Consequently, there is less reinnervation in more distal muscles (Fig. 2).

A final muscle power in major proximal muscles of MRC grade 4/5 was noted only in patients who had been operated on within a month or earlier after the trauma. Two cases of obstetrical brachial plexus lesion with root avulsion were subjected to reimplantation surgery (Carlstedt *et al.* 2000). There was a delay to surgery of more than 6 months; consequently, the functional outcome was equivocal.

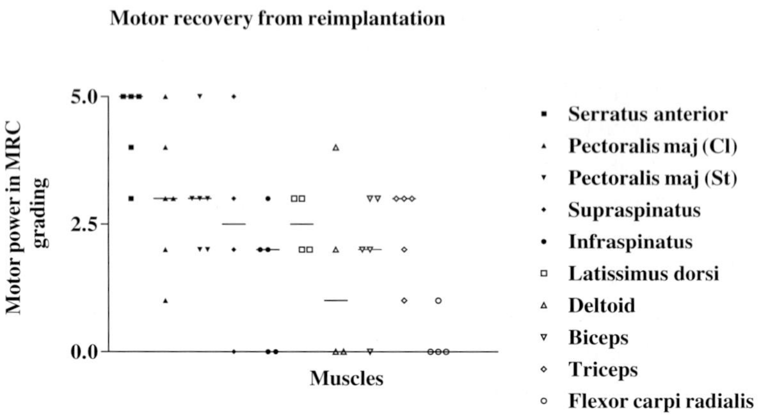

Fig. 2 Recovery of muscle power after spinal cord reconnection of avulsed ventral roots. Power decreases in distal direction.

Patients who were operated on late recovered very little or gained only nonuseful muscle power. This is consistent with the experimental findings of motoneuron loss after avulsion injury depending on the loss of connection with the periphery and its neurotrophic influence causing apoptotic motoneuron death, as well as excitotoxicity by ischemic cell death (Bergerot *et al.* 2004). Moreover, motoneuron programs for repair are available for a limited period after injury and are effective only if the severed axons are offered a conduit for regrowth (Gordon *et al.* 2003). When reconstruction is delayed, the growth-associated genes are downregulated and the neurons become atrophic or die. With delay of repair, there is also an impairment of Schwann cell ability to support regeneration (Sulaiman *et al.* 2002) and a deterioration of the denervated muscles (Gordon *et al.* 2003) (see Chap. 6). In spite of a considerable motoneuron loss from the root avulsion trauma, there was a consistent recovery of muscle power, which was near to normal in proximal muscle groups. The ability of surviving motoneurons to establish larger than normal motor units which can compensate for an 80% loss of neurons is obviously of importance in this recovery (Gordon *et al.* 1993).

Magnetic cortical stimulation demonstrated and verified the clinical observation of connectivity from motor cortex to the previously denervated muscles through the reconstructed spinal cord–peripheral nerve trajectories. The latency of the muscle response was generally longer than in the intact arm, indicating that the regenerated nerve fibres were not fully developed and less myelinated than on the normal side (Fig. 3).

The typical outcome of the reimplantation of three or four ventral roots, or from peripheral nerve grafts to the pertinent avulsed spinal cord segments in adult patients, is recovery of function in shoulder and proximal arm muscles for elbow function. Occasional activity in one or two muscles distal to the elbow, like the brachioradial or pronator muscles, was noted; but distal muscles, like the intrinsics in the hand, were not reinnervated. This is not surprising, as a similar outcome of a proximal median or ulnar nerve lesion can be expected. This is likely to depend on a defective neurotrophic axonal guidance to the appropriate distal targets in time (Brushart 1988; Brushart 1993; Gordon *et al.* 2003). Aberrant muscle reinnervation is therefore likely to result in no or poor function in the hand. In a preadolescent boy who had sustained a complete plexus avulsion injury, spinal cord reimplantation, however, resulted in recovered hand function together with useful activity in shoulder and arm (see below) (Carlstedt *et al.* 2004).

In the majority of cases, recovery of proximal arm function is of great value for the patient, as in several cases after root reimplantation the patients could use their injured arm as a support together with the uninjured arm (see Fig. 1). This recovery of function, as found in long-term follow-up studies, is of the same magnitude as the result of repair of ruptured C5, C6, or upper trunk, or as the result of nerve transfers (Fig. 4).

The functional outcome or use of the arm as assessed by the Narakas score after ventral root–spinal cord reimplantation is in line with the outcome of repair of upper brachial plexus rupture with avulsion of roots C7–T1. From reimplanting the upper brachial plexus ventral roots, the devastating and most severe complete C5–T1 avulsion injury becomes "upgraded" to a less severe type

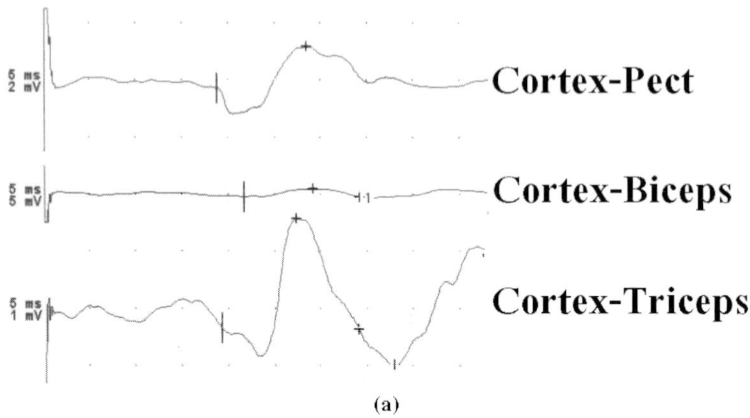

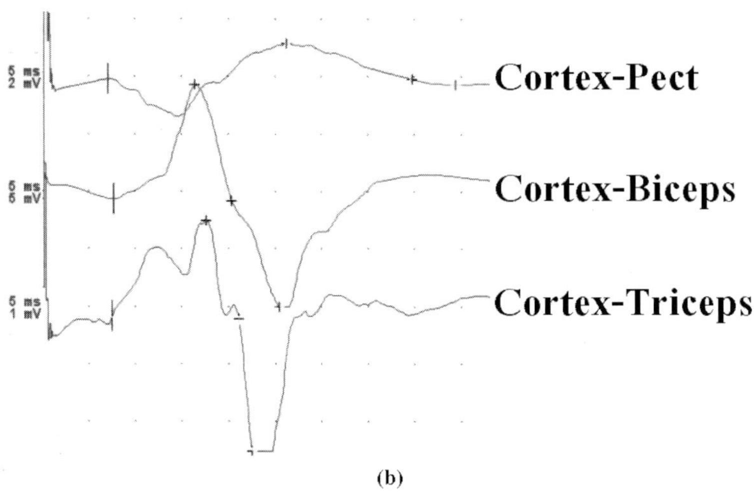

Fig. 3 Motor responses from transcranial magnetic stimulation in a case of complete brachial plexus avulsion. (a) Affected arm; (b) Normal arm. Note the reduced amplitude and increased latency of the motor response in the affected arm (from Htut *et al.* 2007).

of injury consisting of upper plexus nerve ruptures and lower root avulsions (Fig. 5).

Severe cocontractions or synkineses between agonistic and antagonistic muscles occurred in most patients (Fig. 6). For instance, there was a long-standing presence of cocontractions between biceps

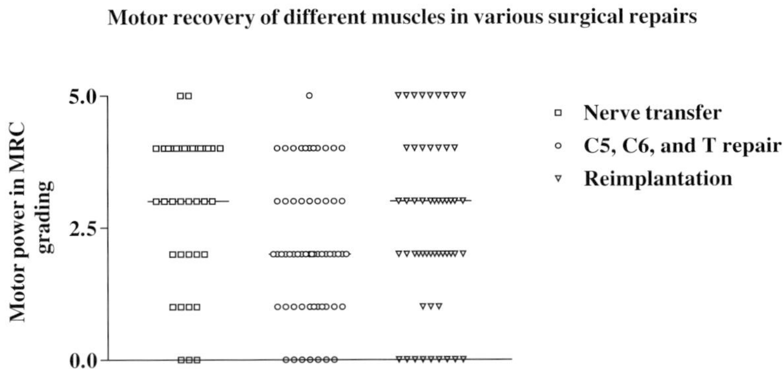

Fig. 4 There is no statistically significant difference in motor recovery from reimplantation versus nerve transfers ($P = 0927$); but there is a significant difference between nerve transfer and C5, C6, or upper trunk repair ($P = 0088$) (Mann–Whitney U test).

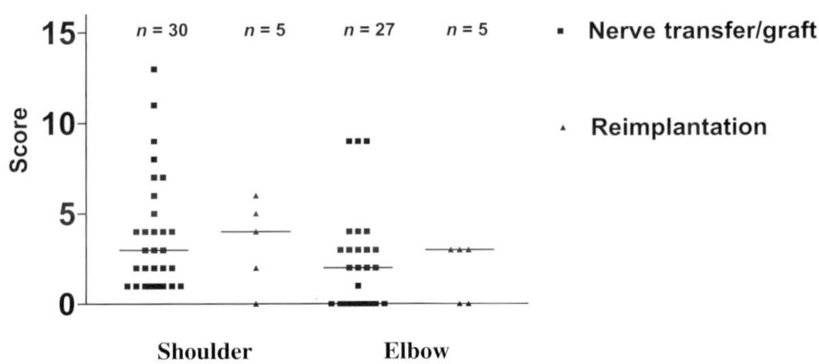

Fig. 5 There is no statistically significant difference in the Narakas score of shoulder ($P = 0.9436$) and elbow ($P = 0.9792$) between patients repaired by means of reimplantation and other surgical repairs (Mann–Whitney U test).

and triceps on both flexion and extension. This is in accordance with the animal experiments showing a nonspecific recruitment of motoneurons to reinnervate pertinent muscles; the lack of guidance of nerve regeneration causes aberrant muscle reinnervation. In previous primate studies, a random reinnervation of arm muscles from the normally discrete and topographically arranged populations of motoneurons in the ventral horn of the spinal cord was demonstrated (Hallin *et al.* 1999). From the normal somatotopographic

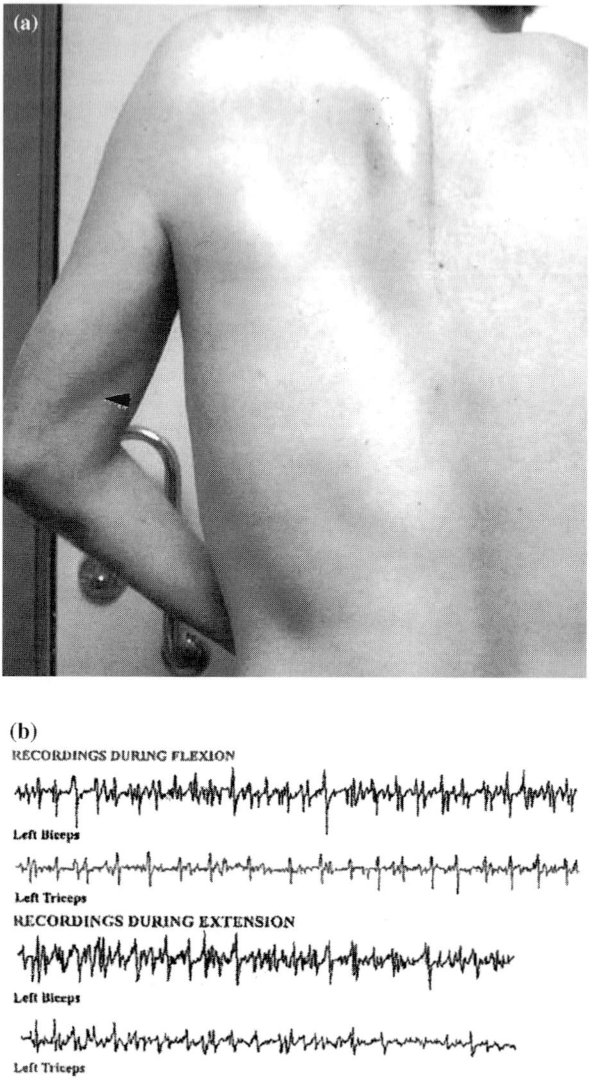

Fig. 6 (a) Synkinesis with widespread activity in the shoulder. (b) Simultaneous surface electrode recordings obtained from antagonistic muscles reinnervated after spinal cord implantation of avulsed ventral roots. Cocontractions occurred in both muscles on flexion as well as extension movements of the elbow (Carlstedt *et al.* 2000).

organisation of motoneurons in the ventral horn, different functional types of nerve cells had extended processes into the implanted ventral root. Judging by their position in the ventral horn, neurons that normally innervate trunk muscles or antagonistic muscles such as the triceps muscle participated in reinnervation of the biceps muscle. Functionally, this deficient specificity of muscle reinnervation was revealed in the experimental animals by means of retrograde labelling and, clinically as well as electrophysiologically, as cocontractions (Hallin *et al.* 1999). Reimplantation of the avulsed ventral root or a PNS graft to the spinal cord attracts any motoneuron in the adjacent segment of the ventral horn to extend new axons into the introduced growth-promoting PNS conduit. As the new axons elongate along the peripheral nerves, there is no direction of growth to the appropriate muscle target, but muscle reinnervation is more or less a random process. Synkinesis is also possible as a result of several axons being produced by the same motoneuron (Havtorn and Kellerth 1987).

Biceps and triceps were usually involved in cocontractions that were elicited by volitional limb movements and disturbed full use of the arm (Fig. 6). The recruitment of nonspecific motoneurons to reinnervate a particular muscle seemed beneficial, as power was always better in muscles with synkinesis than without (Fig. 7). This indicates that the conditions for regeneration of muscle function are better when there is synkinesis, but there is an unspecific recruitment of motoneurons for reinnervation.

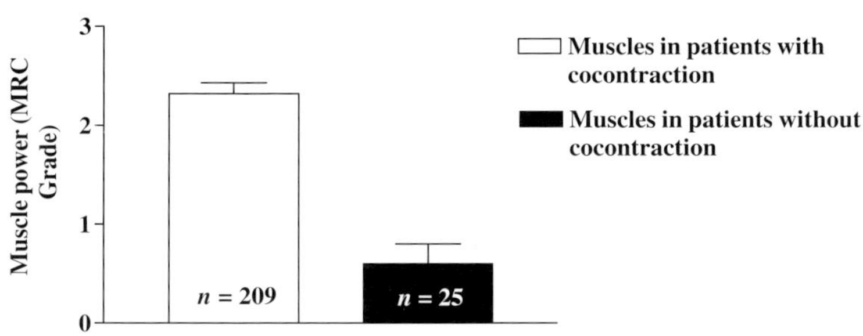

Fig. 7 Regenerated power in muscles with and without synkinesis after spinal cord reconnection to avulsed ventral roots.

There was an eventual tendency for one of the antagonistic muscles — the biceps or the triceps — to dominate and for the other to be functionally suppressed, indicating a degree of plasticity. After approximately 2 years, acceptable dexterity with adequate movements had been achieved, but isolated contraction of individual muscles still could not be performed.

Inappropriate muscle reinnervation also applies to the phrenic motoneurons, regenerating to arm muscles after reimplantation of ventral root or PNS graft, causing respiratory-related limb muscle contractions. This peculiar type of synergism was noted in some patients, where the implantation into the C5 spinal cord segment provoked spontaneous contractions of arm muscles in synchrony with respiration, i.e. "the breathing arm" phenomenon (Swift 1994). Muscle contractions synchronous with spontaneous inspiration were generally related to recovery of volitional function, but could also occur in muscles without voluntary function, i.e. MRC 0/5. Different combinations of muscles, mainly in the C5 myotome (i.e. pectoral, deltoid, biceps, and triceps muscles), showed this activity (Fig. 8).

The breathing arm phenomenon could occur together with antagonistic muscle synkinesis, i.e. cocontractions between biceps and triceps. However, there was respiratory-driven activity only in one of those muscles. There was no correlation between muscle power and the occurrence of breathing arm.

Elbow flexion from respiratory-induced arm muscle contractions has been described as resulting from regeneration within the PNS in patients who have had nerve transfers because of severe brachial plexus injuries, particularly transfers of intercostal nerves (Malessy *et al.* 1998). However, the occurrence of this phenomenon in patients after complete brachial plexus avulsion injury with subsequent spinal cord reimplantation is caused by CNS or spinal cord regeneration. The anatomical background to this phenomenon is that the caudal part of the phrenic motoneuron nucleus is extending into the C5 segment. These neurons are situated most medially in the ventral horn and, after reimplantation of an avulsed ventral root or a peripheral nerve conduit into this segment, phrenic motoneurons

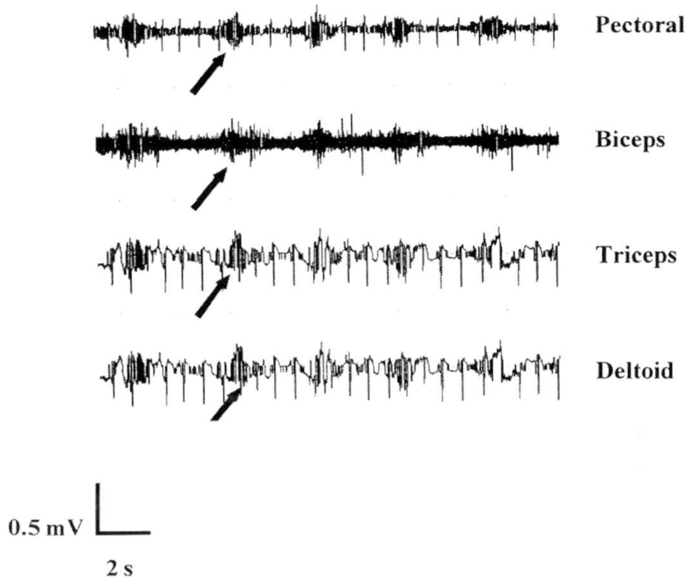

Fig. 8 Multichannel EMG recording of muscles showing bursts of motor units firing synchronously with inspiration (from Carlstedt *et al.* 2004).

are recruited to extend axons along the peripheral nerves to the arm rather than into the phrenic nerve to the diaphragm (Fig. 9).

Synkinesis and the breathing arm phenomenon were noted in long-term follow-up examinations, indicating a stationary condition without any signs of correction over time. This is in contrast to the spontaneous muscle activity occurring after peripheral nerve transfers that eventually disappeared and was followed by volitional control and endurance, which improved and became quite satisfactory over several years (Friedman *et al.* 1990; Chuang *et al.* 1992; Nagano *et al.* 1992; Narakas and Hentz 1988). In those cases, compensatory mechanisms in supraspinal centres were described to correct the respiratory-driven spontaneous activity (Mano *et al.* 1995; Malessey *et al.* 1998). In general, there was no sign of spinal cord plasticity to modulate muscle activity to become purely voluntary. The lack of plasticity, as well as methods to correct the misdirection of motoneurons, is also known from cases of children with obstetrical brachial

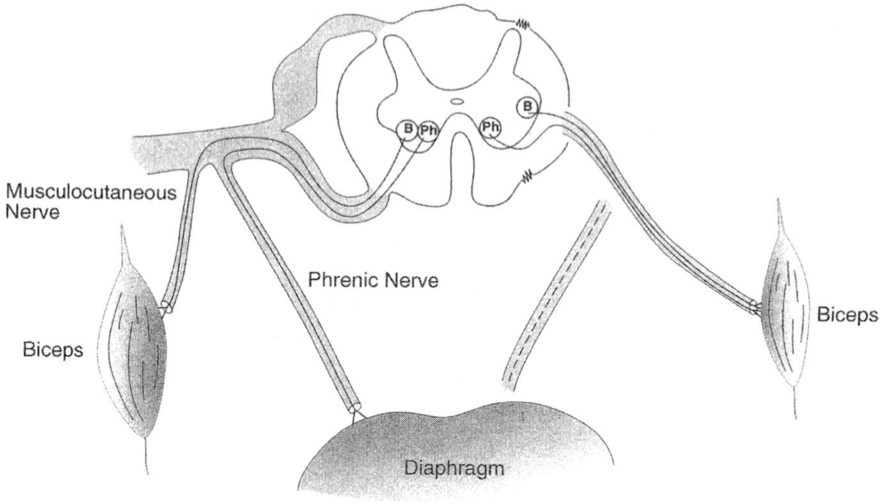

Fig. 9 Diagram showing erroneous spinal cord regeneration of axons from the phrenic motoneuron nucleus in the cervical spinal cord, causing the "breathing arm" phenomenon. Ph, phrenic motoneurons; B, biceps motoneurons.

plexus injury (Roth 1983). In experimental studies, this lack of modification of inappropriately connected spinal motoneurons has been documented, even in the young or immature animal (Gordon *et al.* 1986).

Sensory recovery

Sensory recovery is poor after this type of surgery, where only motor conduits have been reconstructed (Htut *et al.* 2006). In contrast to motor recovery, sensation was always worse in segments affected by root avulsion than spinal nerve rupture. Pinprick sensation was usually subnormal in C5, diminished in C6, and absent in C7–T1. Joint position sense could be appreciated at the shoulder, but also at the elbow. The return of some sensory functions such as proprioception temperature and pain in avulsed dermatomes is unexpected and difficult to explain, as only the ventral roots have been reconnected to the pertinent spinal cord segments. Whether this function depends on extensions of new processes from dorsal horn neurons

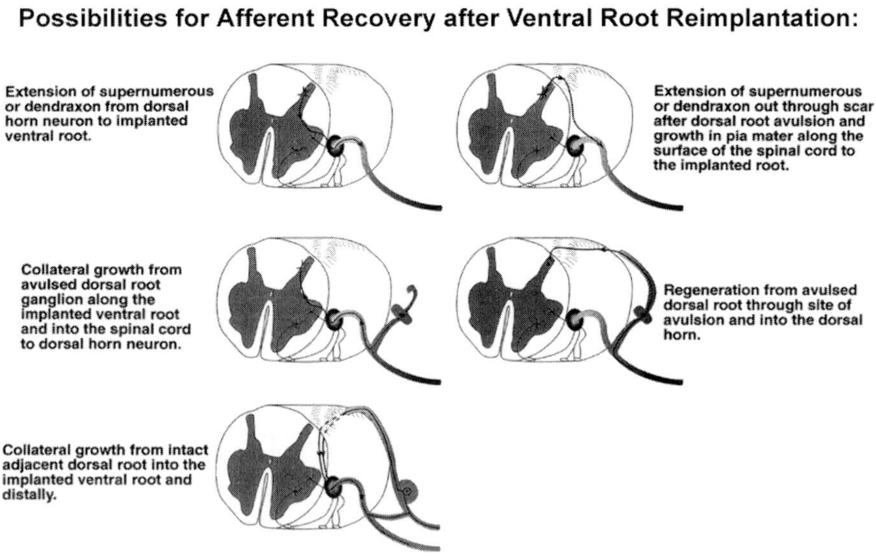

Fig. 10 Some possibilities of sprouting from dorsal horn neurons to reach the periphery.

along the implanted ventral root, or whether it is related to collaterals from adjacent levels, is at present unknown (Fig. 10).

Sensory stimulation within the avulsed dermatomes was mostly perceived abnormally and/or experienced at remote sites as referred sensation (Htut *et al.* 2006). Intraspinal afferent sprouting, producing terminal fields extending into spinal cord segments that have sustained root avulsion and deafferentation (McMahon and Kett-White 1991), could explain such a phenomenon as referrals of sensation from the region of the neck to the hand or vice versa. Classical "right way" referral of sensation — when sensory stimulation of the hand was perceived at the trunk, neck or face — or "wrong way" referral of sensation — from the face, neck, or trunk to the affected arm — occurred (Berman *et al.* 1998; Kew *et al.* 1997). In the early weeks after injury and repair, there was referral of sensation from central parts of the body, even viscera, to the affected arm; but persistent "wrong way" referral of sensation from the region of the intercostal nerve territory to the arm appeared much later, as did the "right way" referral of sensation.

The "right way" of referral of sensation appears as an early sign of recovery, for instance, after nerve transfer (Chuang *et al.* 1992). Following such procedures, sensory stimuli delivered to the recipient site are referred to the donor site. As this can be a consistent perception in many cases, it seems as if cortical circuits within the somatosensory system are not easily corrected for deafferentation and eventually misdirect ional growth of sensory fibres. The "wrong way" referral of sensation, on the other hand, indicates plasticity rather than recovery. This is obvious in patients who, even a long time after surgery, have not developed sensation in the hand; but who perceive sensation in the hand when the neck, trunk, or face is touched. This phenomenon could occur early after the injury, suggesting unmasking of pre-existing connections (Borsook *et al.* 1998). Intracortical sprouting could be the reason for the later-appearing "wrong way referral of sensation" (Kaas *et al.* 1983).

Not all patients experienced referral of sensation. It appeared that those who did not have referral of sensation within some time after injury and repair would not in the future have such an experience. This phenomenon usually changed with time in terms of intensity of sensation and could gradually fade away.

In contrast to the lack of sensory recovery in adult patients with complete brachial prexus injury is the observation of excellent sensory return in the majority of children after obstetric complete brachial plexus injury with multiple root avulsions, having good localisation of touch and no referral of sensation (Anand and Birch 2002).

After repair of a peripheral nerve to a muscle or a nerve transfer, there is some reinnervation of mechanoreceptors, such as muscle spindles, by large rapidly conducting afferent fibres (group I or II) (Sai *et al.* 1996). However, reinnervated muscles, even after a peripheral nerve injury and repair, suffer a massive reduction in afferent reinnervation with various kinds of abnormally responsive afferents (Banks *et al.* 1985). The ability to recover a central nervous control over reinnervated muscles is usually disappointing. The lack of sensory reconnection with the pertinent spinal cord segment after intraspinal repair means lack of muscle proprioception.

A mass movement without the ability to activate individual joints is a sign of supraspinal-led activity without proprioceptive feedback. To some extent, this deficient afferent control over muscle function leads to cocontractions. Some degree of muscle proprioception would be necessary for good muscle function. The role of afferent feedback control has been questioned, however. The central motor program alone may be sufficient to execute learned simple movements such as elbow flexion. Nevertheless, the afferent feedback system is essential when movements involve small, precise contractions, such as intrinsic hand muscle function (Gandevia and Burke 1994; Wolpert *et al.* 1995).

Limb function, and in particular purposeful movements, have been described in a rare example of sensory neuropathy with loss of muscle afferents (Cole and Sedgwick 1992). The patients could learn to compensate for the loss of perception of muscle function or movements with other sensory inputs, such as vision, and they could locomote themselves and move inside and outside their own personal space (Cole 1995; Cole and Paillard 1995). Hand function is possible without sensation, but there is no dexterity (Rothwell *et al.* 1982).

Nevertheless, the original concept established by Sherrington (1894) that muscle function is not possible without sensory function has been revised, as there are now laboratory and patient studies that have shown otherwise. For instance, an acute sensory neuropathy (a cross-reaction between an antibody raised to an infection and the large sensory myelinated neurons in the dorsal root ganglia) leaves the patient permanently without the perception of touch and movement or joint position sense below the neck (Sterman *et al.* 1980). About a dozen such subjects have been described. They have recovered motor functions to a varying degree, according to the level at which the neuropathy starts, the age at onset of disease, and possibly each subject's commitment to learning to move under cognitive and visual control.

This rare neuropathy allows some physiological observations on the mechanisms of sensation without large myelinated sensory contribution. Electrical and laser-induced evoked potentials have been recorded (Cole and Katifi 1991). It has become obvious from such studies that patients with this sensory deficit had managed to re-establish some limited and partially noncognitive motor programs (Cole and Sedgwick 1992; Lajoie *et al.* 1996). The discrimination of peripherally held weights (Fleury *et al.* 1995) and the programming of movement in the absence of peripheral feedback (Miall *et al.* 1995) have allowed observations on the sense of effort, motor memory, and endpoint versus force/amplitude models of movement (Blouin *et al.* 1996; Vercher *et al.* 1996; Vercher *et al.* 1997), and have increased our understanding of the way in which the central motor control is coded.

Pain

The severe pain sustained by patients suffering from brachial plexus injury is typical (Frazier and Skillern 1911; Htut *et al.* 2006), and is presumed to be caused by the generation of abnormal activity in deafferented spinal cord segments (Ovelmen-Levitt 1988). There is a correlation between the number of roots avulsed and the severity of pain (Htut *et al.* 2006). Recently, a description of pain alleviation after transfers of nerves to the avulsed brachial plexus was given (Berman *et al.* 1998; Htut *et al.* 2006). However, what is remarkable is that, in patients with complete avulsion injury to the brachial plexus followed by ventral root reimplantation, the reduction of pain is correlated to the return of muscle activity rather than other qualities of function (Berman *et al.* 1998). There is no relationship between alleviation of pain and referral of sensation, although both phenomena are thought to be due to plasticity in the central nervous system (Htut *et al.* 2006). It is possible that reorganisation after deafferentation is widely spread and probably involves bilateral cerebral structures (Kaas *et al.* 1983).

In patients whose recovery of motor function was limited to the upper part of the extremity, there is persistent pain in the hand. In the case of a preadolescent boy with complete plexus avulsion, there was recovery in all parts of the arm and the hand after reimplantation, and there was consequently complete alleviation of the severe postinjury pain when motor function recovered (see case below). The mechanism behind this is difficult to explain, but it is known that selective loss of motor fibres after ventral rhizotomy can provoke pain in animals (Sheth *et al.* 2002; Wu *et al.* 2002) and man (Ali *et al.* 2002). Cortical reorganisation has been correlated with severity of neuropathic pain (Flor *et al.* 1995). Successful motor recovery could lead to the re-establishment of normal inhibitory processes, reverting the cortical process leading to pain.

In some patients, there was allodynia to mechanical and/or thermal stimulation (Htut *et al.* 2006). The area of allodynia was at the border zone of affected and unaffected dermatomes, usually at the border of T1 and T2 dermatomes, at the back of the elbow. The allodynia was not bothersome and was minor in comparison with the deafferentation pain. This condition could depend on abnormally sensitised peripheral nociceptic fibres that induce secondary changes in reorganisation of the dorsal horn and central processing, leading to spinal cord hyperexcitability and allodynia (Baron 2000a; Baron 2000b). The intact nociceptors of the adjacent uninjured spinal nerves may acquire abnormal spontaneous activity, and chemical sensitivity may play a role in creating or maintaining an abnormal pain state (Campbell 2001; Wu *et al.* 2002).

Remarkably, there is no pain or neuropathic syndromes in neonates after the same type of brachial plexus injuries (Anand and Birch 2002). Sprouting and/or maturation of descending inhibitory tracts, i.e. CNS plasticity which is more pronounced in the immature individual, may account for the absence of the devastating root avulsion pain in young children.

Illustrative cases of recovery after total brachial plexus avulsion and reimplantation

Case 1: WH. The entire plexus had been reconnected to the spinal cord by reimplantation into segments C5, C6, C7, and C8. Muscle recovery started after about 8–10 months, at the shoulder and elbow. Two years postoperatively, there was normal power (5/5) in the trapezius and serratus anterior muscles. Subnormal power (4/5) was noted in the deltoid and biceps muscles as well as in forearm, wrist, and finger flexors. There was some function (1–2/5) in triceps and intrinsic hand muscles, and no clinical function in wrist and finger extensors. Hand function with the ability to perform a grasp and make a fist had recovered 3 years after surgery (Fig. 11). There were severe cocontractions among all muscles (see below), as well as respiratory-induced contractions among proximal arm muscles (see Table 1).

There were perceptions of touch, proprioception, and vibration in the shoulder and elbow; but no sensation in the distal part of the arm and hand. There was no pseudomotor function in the hand. Touching the ipsilateral clavicular region was perceived into the hand as "wrong way" referred sensation.

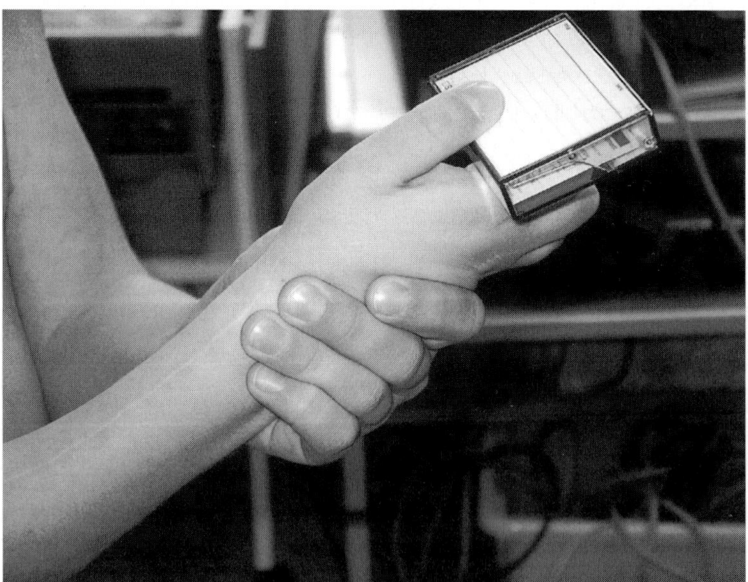

Fig. 11 Case WH. Three years after complete C5–T1 left-sided brachial plexus avulsion injury in a 9-year-old boy. All parts of the brachial plexus are reconnected to the spinal cord. There is return of arm function, but without extensor activity. There is a pinch grip from restored intrinsic function, but the wrist needs to be stabilised due to absent extensor function.

Table 1 Follow-up muscle power in MRC grades. The occurrence of cocontractions (c) and breathing arm activity (b) is indicated.

Patient	Muscle Power								
	Pect C5–T1	Delt, SS C5	LD C6, C7	Biceps C6	Triceps C6, C7	FCR C6, C7	FCU C7, C8	FDP C8, T1	ADM T1
WH	5_{cb}	5	4_{cb}	4_{cb}	1_{cb}	3	4_{cb}	4_{cb}	1_{cb}
JJ	5_{b}	5		4_{cb}	3_{c}	1			

Pain was initially located to the entire extremity, and was treated with 1600 mg of gabapentin without complete resolution of pain. In conjunction with return of motor function, starting about 8–10 months after surgery, pain disappeared completely.

Electromyography showed good recruitment of motor units in pectorals, deltoid, triceps, biceps, wrist and finger flexors, and intrinsic muscles of the hand (adductor digiti minimi, ADM). There were cocontractions in all muscles and inspiratory-provoked muscle activity in biceps, triceps, deltoid, and pectoral muscles (Fig. 8).

Electromagnetic cortical stimulation produced muscle responses in all of the above muscles with somewhat prolonged latency and smaller amplitude, except in the pectoral muscle, which had a higher amplitude compared to the intact side (Fig. 3).

Case 2: JJ. The spinal cord segments C5, C6, and C7 were reconnected to the upper and middle trunks of the plexus by reimplantation. Functional return started about 10 months postoperatively among proximal arm muscles. Three years after surgery, there was normal power in pectoral and shoulder muscles. Subnormal power in elbow flexion and extension was noted (Fig. 12). There was subclinical activity (1/5) in flexor carpi radialis (FCR). There were cocontractions between biceps and triceps. Inspiratory-related contractions in the pectoral and biceps muscles were noted (see Table 1).

Sensation of touch was limited to the shoulder and upper medial part of the arm, i.e. C5 and Th2, with normal perception of joint position in the shoulder and some joint sensation in the elbow. There was no sensation distal to the elbow and no pseudomotor function

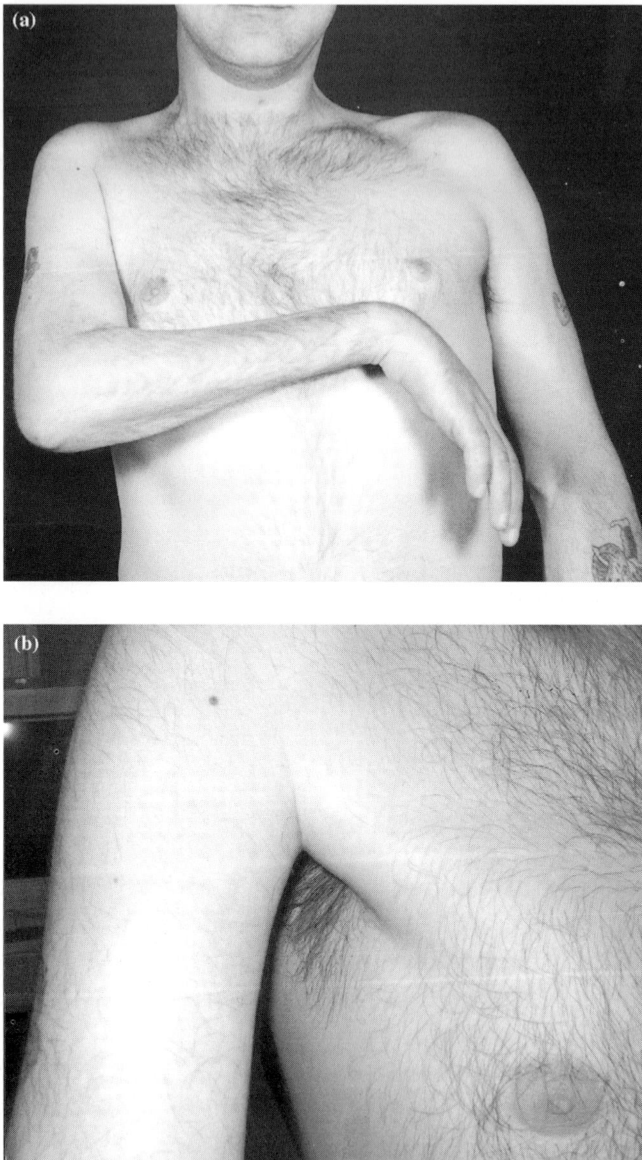

Fig. 12 Case JJ. Same injury as in Fig. 11. (a) Restored function in shoulder and upper arm with elbow flexion 3 years after complete brachial plexus avulsion and spinal cord reimplantation. No wrist and hand function. (b) Activity in the sternal part of the pectoral muscle indicates a nondirectional reinnervation from the upper part of the brachial plexus. (c) An MRI of the C6 spinal cord segment 3 years after reimplantation surgery.

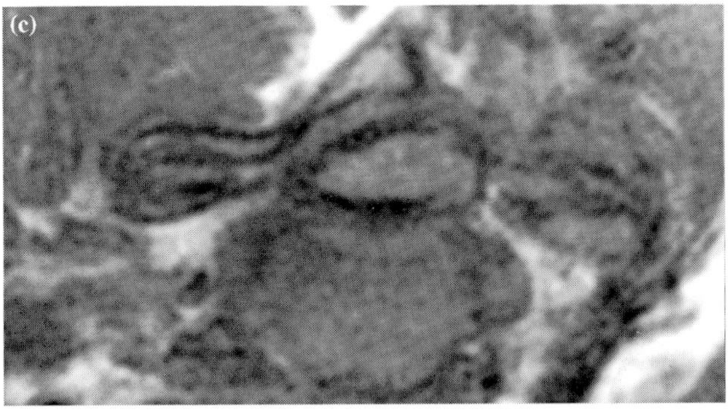

Fig. 12 (*Continued*)

in the hand. There was a constant pain, with excruciating burning and pulsing pain in the hand.

Electromyography showed no muscle unit potential (MUP) in deltoid or biceps muscles 6 months postsurgery. At 3 years after surgery, there were normal-looking MUPs on voluntary contraction in the biceps and pectoral, as well as small but normal-looking MUPs on voluntary contraction in the deltoid, triceps, infraspinatus, and long flexors of the forearm. There were cocontractions between biceps, triceps, and pectoral muscles. Normal inspiration elicited MUPs in the deltoid, triceps, and biceps. This muscle activity was not strong enough to produce movements.

Electromagnetic stimulation produced muscle responses in biceps and pectoral muscles of reduced amplitude and somewhat longer latency than on the intact side. MRI showed signs of previous root avulsions and reimplantation (Fig. 12).

It is remarkable to observe that the reduction in pain is correlated to the return of muscle activity rather than other qualities of function (Berman *et al.* 1998). This concept is certainly supported in the present study, where the patient WH — who recovered muscle activity in all parts of his upper extremity, but very limited sensory function — experienced a complete alleviation of his severe post-injury pain when muscle function regenerated. In contrast, the other patient (JJ), who had motor recovery only proximal to the elbow, is still suffering from excruciating pain in his hand, where there has been no recovery.

The present report of two cases of complete C5–Th1 brachial plexus avulsion from the spinal cord demonstrates clinically and by means of different electrophysiological techniques (EMG, TMS) the efficacy of spinal cord reimplantation surgery. Most important is the alleviation of pain followed by this treatment. The regeneration of motor function into the hand demonstrates the potential of this approach in bringing the reconstructed neural networks close to an original status rather than palliative function through remote compensatory mechanisms. To further improve the functional outcome of this spinal cord surgery with the application of pharmaceutical compounds and growth factors is an obvious and immediate objective.

Lumbosacral Plexus

Return of function after intraspinal repair is slow, with the best outcome occurring for the proximal muscles and to a lesser extent for calf muscles (Table 2). The basic requirements for standing and walking are hip and knee stability and flexion. These key functions depend on sufficient power in proximal muscles such as the iliopsoas, the quadriceps, and the glutei muscles. In patients who had been unable to stand or walk without support due to paralysis of those muscles from sacral nerve root ruptures, intraspinal surgery resulted in independent locomotion.

Illustrative cases

Case 3. A 29-year-old man had sustained sacral fractures through the sacral foramina with loss of motor function distal to the knee. Scanning demonstrated pseudomeningoceles at S1–S3 foramina. A laminectomy revealed ruptures of S1–S3 roots.

Nine months after intraspinal reconstruction of the ruptured roots S1–S3, there was some return of muscle function in the gastrocnemius and tibialis anterior muscles. At 1.5 years postoperatively,

Table 2 Outcome and surgical treatments after intraspinal sacral plexus injuries.

Case	Surgery Delay	Procedure	Outcome
1	11 months	Graft S2–Sup Glut N	Hip stability and movements
2	12 months	Repair S1–S3 Roots	Recovery of ankle movements
3	4 days	Repair S1–S3 Roots	Recovery of ankle movements
4	8 months	Grafts S1,S2–Sup Glut N	Hip stability and movements
5	3 months	Grafts L5, S1, S2–Sacral plex.	Hip, knee, ankle movements

the triceps surae muscle strength was 3/5 and that of the tibialis anterior 2/5 (Fig. 13).

Case 4. A 22-year-old woman had sustained a complicated pelvic fracture with dissociation of sacroiliac joints; and had lost function in hip extensor muscles, hamstrings, and muscles distal to the knee, i.e. a sacral plexus lesion. Intraspinal lesions of L5 to S2 were diagnosed. After a laminectomy, the proximal stumps of S1 and S2 could be found. By sural nerve grafts, those roots were reconnected to the gluteal nerves.

About 1 year after surgery, she was able to walk without support with a small limp. There had been a recovery in glutei muscles up to 3/5. Electrophysiology demonstrated reinnervation. Power in hip muscles improved, but not in the leg.

Case 5. A 3-year-old girl who had been hit by a car had sustained severe pelvic and internal organ injuries. She had lost function in the right leg and was unable to walk. There was an intraspinal lesion to the sacral plexus that was verified by electrophysiology and myelography. An intraspinal repair by means of sural nerve grafts from the proximal nerve root stumps to the distally displaced sacral plexus was done.

Within 6 months after the repair, there was some slight recovery of glutei and hamstring function. Electrophysiological signs of

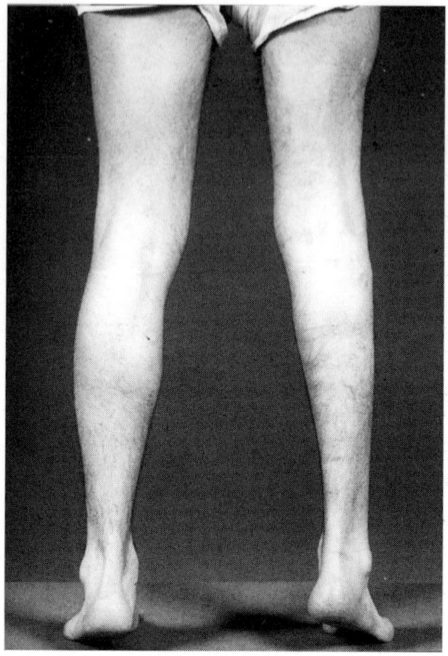

Fig. 13 Outcome from intrapelvic reconstruction of a right-sided lumbosacral plexus injury. Recovery of proximal leg and and some calf muscles has occurred, enabling the patient to stand on his toes (Lang *et al.* 2004).

recovery in calf muscles were noted 9 months after the repair. Three years later, she was followed up independently, as she had moved with her family to another country. A limb length discrepancy was noted. There was 4/5 muscle power in the hip muscles and hamstring muscles, but only slight reinnervation in muscles below the knee. There was neuropathic pain in the distal part of the leg.

In cases of proximal or intraspinal ruptures where the proximal root stumps cannot be retrieved, nerve transfers are possible and can mean definite improvement in function, independence, and quality of life (see Chap. 5).

Conclusion

The best outcome from intraspinal repair and spinal cord reimplantation is seen when the surgery is performed in connection with the trauma. The magnitude of restored function is the same as when ruptured spinal nerves in the plexus have been reconstructed. Proximal arm and shoulder muscles recover the strongest muscle power, but there is synkinesis among those well-recovered muscles that disturbs the functional outcome. Antagonistic muscle cocontractions inspiratory and induced muscle contractions, the so-called "breathing arm" phenomenon, occur in many patients. Recovery of distal or intrinsic hand function is possible. Pain is alleviated in parallel with the return of muscle activity. Sensory function is present at best as referred perception, probably through collaterals or central plasticity. The relationship between plastic changes occurring in the nervous system after deafferentation, i.e. dorsal root avulsion injury, and neuropathic pain seems complex, but an understanding of these mechanisms will help to develop treatment programs in order to improve the management of chronic neuropathic pain.

References

Ali Z, Meyer RA, Belzberg AJ, Neuropathic pain after C7 spinal nerve transection in man, *Pain* **96**:41–47, 2002.

Anand P, Birch R, Restoration of sensory function and lack of long-term chronic pain syndromes after brachial plexus injury in human neonates, *Brain* **125**:113–122, 2002.

Banks RW, Barker D, Brown HG, Sensory reinnervation of muscles following nerve section and suture in cats, *J Hand Surg* **10**:340–344, 1985.

Baron R, Neuropathic pain. The long path from mechanisms to mechanism-based treatment, *Anaesthesist* **49**:373–386, 2000a.

Baron R, Peripheral neuropathic pain: from mechanisms to symptoms, *Clin J Pain* **16**:S12–S20, 2000b.

Bergerot A, Shortland PJ, Anand P *et al.*, Co-treatment with riluzole and GDNF is necessary for functional recovery after ventral root avulsion injury, *Exp Neurol* **187**:359–366, 2004.

Berman JS, Birch R, Anand P, Pain following human brachial plexus injury with spinal cord root avulsion and the effect of surgery, *Pain* **75**:199–207, 1998.

Blouin J, Gauthier GM, Vercher JL, Cole JD, The relative contribution of retinal and extraretinal signals in determining the accuracy of reaching movements in normal subjects and a deafferented patient, *Exp Brain Res* **109**:148–153, 1996.

Borsook D, Becerra L, Fishman S *et al.*, Acute plasticity in the human somatosensory cortex following amputation, *Neuroreport* **9**:1013–1017, 1998.

Brushart TM, Preferential reinnervation of motor nerves by regenerating motor axons, *J Neurosci* **8**:1026–1031, 1988.

Brushart TM, Motor axons preferentially reinnervate motor pathways, *J Neurosci* **13**:2730–2738, 1993.

Campbell JN, Nerve lesions and the generation of pain, *Muscle Nerve* **24**:1261–1273, 2001.

Carlstedt T, Anand P, Hallin RG *et al.*, Spinal nerve root repair and reimplantation of avulsed ventral roots into the spinal cord after brachial plexus injury, *J Neurosurg* **93**:237–247, 2000.

Carlstedt T, Anand P, Htut M *et al.*, Restoration of hand function and so called "breathing arm" after intraspinal repair of C5–T1 brachial plexus avulsion injury, *Neurosurg Focus* **16**:article 7, 2004.

Carlstedt T, Grane P, Hallin RG, Noren G, Return of function after spinal cord implantation of avulsed spinal nerve roots, *Lancet* **346**:1323–1325, 1995.

Chuang DC, Yeh MC, Wei FC, Intercostal nerve transfer of the musculocutaneous nerve in avulsed brachial plexus injuries: evaluation of 66 patients, *J Hand Surg [Am]* **14**:822–828, 1992.

Cole JD, *Pride and a Daily Marathon*, MIT Press, Boston, MA, 1995.

Cole JD, Katifi HA, Evoked potentials in a man with a complete large myelinated fibre sensory neuropathy below the neck, *Electroencephalogr Clin Neurophysiol* **80**:103–107, 1991.

Cole JD, Paillard J, Living without touch and peripheral information about body position and movement: studies upon deafferented subjects, in Bermudez J, Marcel A, Eilan N (eds.), *The Body and the Self*, MIT Press, Boston, MA, pp. 245–266, 1995.

Cole JD, Sedgwick EM, The perceptions of force and movement in a man without large myelinated sensory afferents below the neck, *J Physiol* **449**:503–515, 1992.

Cullheim S, Carlstedt T, Risling M, Axon regeneration of spinal motoneurons following a lesion at the cord–ventral root interface: from basic animal research to a new surgical approach in human cases of ventral root avulsion lesions. A review, *Spinal Cord* **37**:811–819, 1999.

Fleury M, Bard C, Teasdale N *et al.*, Weight judgement: the discrimination capacity of a deafferented subject, *Brain* **118**:1149–1156, 1995.

Flor H, Elbert T, Knecht S *et al.*, Phantom-limb pain as a perceptual correlate of cortical reorganization following arm amputation, *Nature* **375**:482–484, 1995.

Frazier CH, Skillern PG, Supraclavicular subcutaneous lesions of the brachial plexus not associated with skeletal injuries, *JAMA* **57**:1957–1963, 1911.

Friedman AH, Nunley JA, Goldner RD *et al.*, Nerve transposition for the restoration of elbow flexion following brachial plexus avulsion injuries, *J Neurosurg* **72**:59–64, 1990.

Gandevia SC, Burke D, Does the nervous system depend on kinesthetic information to control natural limb movements?, in Cordo O, Harnad S (eds.), *Movement Control*, Cambridge University Press, New York, pp. 12–30, 1994.

Gordon T, Stein RB, Thomas CK, Innervation and function of hind-limb muscles in the cat after cross-union of the tibial and peroneal nerves, *J Physiol* **374**:429–441, 1986.

Gordon T, Sulaiman O, Boyd JG, Experimental strategies to promote functional recovery after peripheral nerve injuries, *J Peripher Nerv Syst* **8**:236–250, 2003.

Gordon T, Yang JF, Ayer K *et al.*, Recovery potential of muscle after partial denervation: a comparison between rats and humans, *Brain Res Bull* **30**:477–482, 1993.

Hallin RG, Carlstedt T, Nilsson-Remahl IA, Risling M, Spinal cord implantation of avulsed ventral roots in primates; correlation between restored motor function and morphology, *Exp Brain Res* **124**:304–310, 1999.

Havtorn L, Kellerth JO, Regeneration by supernumerary axons with synaptic terminals in spinal motoneurons of cats, *Nature* **325**:711–714, 1987.

Htut M, Misra P, Anand P *et al.*, Pain phenomena and sensory recovery following brachial plexus avulsion injury and surgical repairs, *J Hand Surg [Br]* **31**:596–605, 2006.

Htut M, Misra P, Anand P *et al.*, Motor recovery and the breathing arm after brachial plexus surgical repairs, including re-implantation of avulsed spinal roots into the spinal cord, *J Hand Surg [Br]* **32**:170–178, 2007.

Kaas JH, Merzenich MM, Killackey HP, The reorganization of somatosensory cortex following peripheral nerve damage in adult and developing mammals. *Annu Rev Neurosci* **6**:325–356, 1983.

Kew JJ, Halligan PW, Marshall JC *et al.*, Abnormal access of axial vibrotactile input to deafferented somatosensory cortex in human upper limb amputees, *J Neurophysiol* **77**:2753–2764, 1997.

Lajoie Y, Teasdale N, Cole JD *et al.*, Gait of a deafferented subject without large myelinated sensory fibers below the neck, *Neurology* **47**:109–115, 1996.

Lang EM, Borges J, Carlstedt T, Surgical treatment of lumbosacral injuries, *J Neurosurg Spine* **1**:64–71, 2004.

Malessy MJ, Thomeer RT, van Dijk JG, Changing central nervous control following intercostal nerve transfer, *J Neurosurg* **89**:568–574, 1998.

Mano Y, Nakamuro T, Tamura R *et al.*, Central motor reorganization after anastomosis of the musculocutaneous and intercostal nerves following cervical root avulsion, *Ann Neurol* **38**:15–20, 1995.

McMahon SB, Kett-White R, Sprouting of peripherally regenerating primary sensory neurones in the adult central nervous system, *J Comp Neurol* **304**:307–315, 1991.

Miall RC, Haggard P, Cole JD, Evidence of a limited visuo-motor memory used in programming wrist movements, *Exp Brain Res* **107**:267–280, 1995.

Nagano A, Ochiai N, Okinaga S, Restoration of elbow flexion in root lesions of brachial plexus injuries, *J Hand Surg [Am]* **17**:815–821, 1992.

Narakas AO, Hentz VR, Neurotization in brachial plexus injuries: indication and results, *Clin Orthop Relat Res* **237**:43–56, 1988.

Ovelmen-Levitt J, Abnormal physiology of the dorsal horn as related to the deafferentation syndrome, *Appl Neurophysiol* **51**:104–116, 1988.

Roth G, Reinnervation dans la paralysie plexulaire brachiale obstetricale, *J Neurol Sci* **58**:103–115, 1983.

Rothwell JC, Traub MM, Day BL *et al.*, Manual motor performance in a deafferented man, *Brain* **105**:515–542, 1982.

Sai K, Kanamaru A, Sibuya M *et al.*, Reconstruction of tonic vibration reflex in the biceps brachii reinnervated by transferred intercostal nerves in patients with brachial plexus injury, *Neurosci Lett* **206**:1–4, 1996.

Sherrington CS, On the anatomical constitution of nerves of skeletal muscles: with remarks on recurrent fibres in the ventral spinal nerve-root, *J Physiol* **17**:211–258, 1894.

Sheth RN, Dorsi MJ, Li Y *et al.*, Mechanical hyperalgesia after an L5 ventral rhizotomy or an L5 ganglionectomy in the rat, *Pain* **96**:63–72, 2002.

Sterman AB, Schaumburg HH, Asbury AK, The acute sensory neuronopathy syndrome: a distinct clinical entity, *Ann Neurol* **7**:354–358, 1980.

Sulaiman OAR, Midha R, Munro CA *et al.*, Chronic Schwann cell denervation and the presence of a sensory nerve reduce motor axonal regeneration, *Exp Neurol* **176**:342–354, 2002.

Swift TR, The breathing arm, *Muscle Nerve* **17**:125–129, 1994.

Vercher JL, Gauthier GM, Cole J, Blouin J, Role of arm proprioception in calibrating the arm–eye temporal coordination, *Neurosci Lett* **237**:109–112, 1997.

Vercher JL, Gauthier GM, Guedon O *et al.*, Self-moved target eye tracing in control and deafferented subjects: roles of arm motor command and proprioception in arm–eye coordination, *J Neurophysiol* **76**:1133–1144, 1996.

Wolpert DM, Ghahramani Z, Jordan MI, An internal model for sensimotor integration, *Science* **269**:1880–1882, 1995.

Wu G, Ringkamp M, Murinson BB, Degeneration of myelinated efferent fibers induces spontaneous activity in uninjured C-fiber afferents, *J Neurosci* **22**:7746–7753, 2002.

9

CONCLUSION

The Future

Spinal cord surgery to restore connectivity after spinal nerve root avulsion injury from traction lesions to the brachial plexus can recover function in the affected arm or even in the hand (Carlstedt *et al.* 2004), alleviate pain, rescue spinal cord nerve cells, and preserve segmental spinal cord circuits. Therefore, this surgical technique is today the most promising treatment in cases of complete brachial plexus avulsion injury (C5–T1). This strategy has encouraging prospects for future treatment of brachial and lumbosacral plexus injuries and possibly of transverse spinal cord injuries, for instance in the conus medullaris.

The recovery of function after avulsion of roots from the spinal cord depends on the findings that some nerve cells (i.e. motoneurons) could survive the trauma, and that their axons (which had been interrupted within the spinal cord white matter) could regrow within the spinal cord as a first and crucial part of the recovery (Carlstedt *et al.* 1986; Cullheim *et al.* 1989). What were original observations in laboratory experiments have taken a long way to become applied in human clinical practice. At present, the shortcomings of this technique are proportionate to the delay of surgery, with death of nerve cells as well as incomplete and unpredictable sensimotor recovery. The outcome of the present surgical strategy for intraspinal plexus lesions is today limited by several conditions:

(1) There is a rapid death of nerve cells after the avulsion trauma.
(2) There is no sensory recovery or afferent feedback.
(3) There is non-specific reinnervation with synergism and deficient hand recovery.

Rapid death of nerve cells after avulsion trauma

There is considerable death among nerve cells after a severe nerve injury, thus obviously interfering with the possibility to restore function by means of surgery. The exact mechanism behind injury-induced neuronal death is not known and appears to be multifactor. Trophic deprivation and glutamate-mediated excitotoxicity can cause ischemic as well as apoptotic cell death. Several substances have been tested and found to curtail neuronal death. Regarding motoneurons, there is a rapid retrograde cell death amounting to about 80% after spinal nerve root avulsion injury. A cascade of molecular events, where glutamate and calcium have been claimed to play major roles in ischemic cell death, follows such injuries. A possibility to maintain motoneurons after such an injury would be to provide antagonists to glutamate release by blocking NMDA receptors, e.g. with riluzole (Doble 1996), and to prevent intracellular overload of calcium by inhibiting L-type voltage-gated calcium channels, e.g. with nimodipine (Mattsson *et al.* 1999).

Motoneurons seem to be highly dependent on interactions with the periphery and supply of trophic molecules, particularly those derived from Schwann cells. This supply is lost after spinal root avulsion injury, which therefore has a detrimental effect on neuron survival through apoptotic cell death. Key trophic factors for both motor and sensory neurons are the brain-derived neurotrophic factor (BDNF) and the glial cell line–derived neurotrophic factor (GDNF). These substances will obviously be supplied "naturally" after reimplantation surgery (Bergerot *et al.* 2004). "Artificial" application of these substances at the avulsion site by osmotic pumps (Li *et al.* 1995), for instance, or directly to the injured motoneurons through the virus vector technique (Blits *et al.* 2004), can rescue motoneurons at least in the short term as well as enhance neurite outgrowth (Novikov *et al.* 1997).

In a recent study, it was shown that a combination of growth factors and substances that inhibits glutamate release, e.g. riluzole, has a most advantageous effect (Bergerot *et al.* 2004). Such a combination will obviously interfere with apoptotic as well as ischemic cell death, but there is also a synergistic effect from the combined treatment with those substances, leading to a persistent amelioration of motoneuron death together with increased synthesis of neurotransmitters — hence, restoration of function. In tests assessing different aspects of recovery, close to normality was noted (Bergerot *et al.* 2004). Single-treatment therapies proved ineffective at rescuing all motoneurons from cell death or at restoring functional recovery. Combination therapies proved to be far more effective and offered a potential new treatment strategy for avulsion-injury patients. In the future, a combination of substances that interferes with apoptotic and necrotic neuronal death as well as augments regeneration is most likely to be used in adults, and is also certainly to be indicated in severe cases of obstetric plexus injury where surgery, for many reasons, must be postponed for some time.

Cell replacement therapy, i.e. to supplement the disappearing or dead neurons with immature cells or undifferentiated cells, can hypothetically augment recovery in cases where neuronal cell death has depleted the motoneuron population. This might appear as the only option, particularly in cases considered for surgery late (over 1 month) after their injury. The use of stem cells for such neuronal replacement therapy, however, remains dubious, although it is possible in culture dishes to direct such undifferentiated cells to show characteristics of motoneurons. Previous experiments where embryonic motoneurons were grafted into the spinal cord showed little signs of integration and functional improvement (Clowry and Vrbova 1992).

No sensory recovery of afferent feedback

It is currently not possible to reconstruct the afferent or sensory pathways, which are obviously necessary for a full recovery. The first part of the regrowing motor axons and the last part of the sensory dorsal root ganglion axons have to negotiate the elongation in the hostile CNS tissue. This is obviously possible to some extent for the motoneuron axons, but not at all for the sensory axons except in cases where growth of dorsal root axons has been reported after NT-3 induced regeneration (Ramer *et al.* 2000; Ramer *et al.* 2001). A major problem is the nonpermissive environment in the spinal cord or CNS to axonal elongation or regrowth after injury. Post-injury cellular response or gial cell scarring and the occurrence of growth-inhibitory substances derived from degrading central nervous myelin, as well as substances such as semaphorins appearing as secreted and membrane-bound proteins, are thought to contribute to this situation (see review by Fawcett and Asher 1999). A specific gene, termed *nogo*, and the proteoglycan NG2 have also been implicated in this process. The role of these molecules is, however, currently revised from being considered exclusively inhibitory to be more of guidance cues or "antiarborisation" substances restricting nerve fibres to particular pathways (Morgenstern *et al.* 2003; Raisman 2003).

The development of molecular biology and the description of various growth-promoting and growth-inhibitory molecules have generally increased the knowledge of subcellular events during nerve injury, degeneration, and regeneration. There has been a great deal of enthusiasm for anticipated improved regeneration of function after injury in the PNS and CNS, applying new molecular therapy derived from these studies. However, there have been little, if any, clinical applications as yet from these endeavours.

In the highly disorganised tissue or scar that follows an injury in the spinal cord or CNS, the experimental strategies to overcome the impediment to regeneration are molecular and cellular strategies, as well as by artificial conduits to bridge the scar region. The use of biochemical agents — including the use of antisense sequences to block the production of the key inhibitory protein and administration of, for instance, chondroitinase enzyme to degrade its functional elements — has been used with some success (Bradbury *et al.* 2002). A possibility to enhance growth within the spinal cord is to offer conduits that are permissive, such as PNS grafts or artificial conduits with qualities that could promote growth. As an artificial conduit, a composite neural guide consisting of a biodegradable carrier (e.g. a soluble glass, with minimal adhesion or fibrosis and full absorption) that contains a microfibrous protein core for cellular-level guidance (e.g. fibronectin) can be used. The effect of the protein-based cell-guidance core has been described (Priestly *et al.* 2002).

The inability of the dorsal root ganglion neurons to negotiate elongation across the PNS–CNS transitional region at the dorsal root–spinal cord junction is notorious (Carlstedt 1985; Ovelmen-Levitt 1988). Efforts to promote sensory regeneration into the spinal cord are still at the experimental stage, as only now do we have a clearer understanding of the mechanisms that limit regeneration in the spinal cord. This has led to strategies that aim to minimise the deleterious effects of trauma and scar formation, or minimise the influence of inhibitory molecules, and maximise and promote trophic support for axonal regeneration by sensory neurons (Priestley *et al.* 2002). An elegant concept is that of cell therapy, which is used to promote the re-establishment of permissive cellular bridges in the spinal cord lesion and thereby create a situation that occurs spontaneously in the peripheral nerve after injury. Experiments with Schwann cells (Li and Raisman 1994), and more successfully with olfactory ensheathing cells (OECs) (Li *et al.* 1997), have resulted in the functional return of lesioned spinal cord tracts (Li *et al.* 2003). Such cells have recently been used for regrowth of dorsal root axons into the spinal cord (Li *et al.* 2004). At the reconstituted dorsal root–spinal cord interface, the OECs formed a ladder-like bridging structure of astrocytic processes, allowing the elongation of dorsal root axons. In addition to the regenerative effect these cells have on the regrowing axons, it was also demonstrated in this study that the OECs are able to reconstruct an anatomical pathway along which the axons can grow. Such reconstruction is a complex histogenetic event requiring the OECs to interact with both Schwann cells of the PNS part of the root and with astrocytes of the spinal cord, forming a tissue bridge along which axons can grow from the severed root into the spinal cord (Li *et al.* 2004). This cellular therapy is possible in cases of dorsal root avulsion injury for recovery of connectivity.

Another, and the most important, consequence of lost sensory connection with the spinal cord is the excruciating pain sustained by patients with root avulsion injury. Pain is proportional to the number of roots avulsed and is considered to depend on spontaneous hyperactivity in spinal cord cells (Guenot *et al.* 2003). Surgical repair strategies that promote functional motor regeneration by means of nerve transfers, as well as by spinal cord reimplantation of avulsed ventral roots, alleviate pain sensation just prior to the onset of voluntary movements (Berman *et al.* 1996; Berman *et al.* 1998; Carlstedt *et al.* 2000). The mechanism underlying pain diminution is unknown, but probably involves CNS plasticity. The pharmacological management of this injury is empirical and there is no current consensus as to how to treat these patients, as the underlying molecular events that occur following avulsion injury are poorly understood.

Several mechanisms may contribute to this pain. Ischemia and excitotoxicity, due to an imbalance of excitatory and inhibitory mechanisms, are likely to be major contributing factors. Degenerating primary afferents will release glutamate and other excitatory transmitters into the extracellular environment, thereby overexciting neurons. Altered levels of voltage-gated sodium channels, which are involved in the generation and propagation of action potentials, are thought to be important, as recent evidence shows that they are upregulated in spinal cord neurons in cases of neuropathic pain after spinal cord injury (Hains *et al.* 2003). Glial cells have recently also been shown to play a role in the production of neuropathic pain. Microglia might induce pain, whilst astrocytes maintain the pain (Watkins and Maier 2003). Substances that interfere with sodium channels inhibiting glutamate release, such as riluzole (Bergerot *et al.* 2004), could be an adjunct to dorsal root reconnection to the spinal cord possibly by cellular treatment for the alleviation of pain.

Nonspecific reinnervation with synergism and deficient hand recovery

There is a lack of direction of growth after all types of nerve surgery, particularly after the most proximal nerve or spinal cord repair. The nerve cells within the spinal cord, if offered a peripheral nerve conduit, will take any opportunity to extend processes and obviously try to reinnervate the first or most proximal target. There is a nonspecific recruitment of spinal cord motoneurons into the implanted PNS graft, for instance phrenic neurons, and there is a tendency to reinnervate the most proximal muscles first. This will obviously result in synergism and hyperreinnervation proximally, but deficient distal reinnervation.

The most conspicuous effects of nondirectional growth of motoneurons after intraspinal repair and spinal cord reimplantation of avulsed ventral roots are the phenomena of "breathing arm" and flexor–extensor muscle cocontraction, which conspire against useful recovery and effective distal limb or hand function. This is an obvious disadvantage, which depends on the nondirectional growth within the PNS rather than on the lack of spinal cord regeneration. Unfortunately, such synkinesis seems today impossible to correct once it is established (Roth 1983). The regeneration of axons into inappropriate pathways is a major contributing factor to the failure of full functional restitution after nerve repair.

In order to augment recovery, guided tissue regeneration is a procedure expected to improve repair. By using biodegradable artificial conduits, axonal regrowth and restoration of nerve trunk continuity is achieved similar to what is seen after an autologous nerve graft, but the outcome is not superior to conventional repair (Giardino *et al.* 1999). Motor recovery, for instance, depends on the accuracy of the direction of growth and reconnection with the original muscles. Factors contributing to a preferential motor reinnervation of motor axons have been described (Brushart and Seiler 1987; Madison *et al.* 1999). Augmentation in the specificity of regeneration has been reported after using electrical current (Al-Majed *et al.* 2000), a technique which also has the advantage of accelerating regrowth. This physical strategy to improve recovery will no doubt be followed in the future by molecular treatments, when more knowledge about specific neuron trophic substances has been achieved.

The root avulsion injury is a limited spinal cord injury that interrupts defined populations of neurons, i.e. the "final common pathway" for motor command and the sensory pathway for the peripheral sensory neurons. Patients with such spinal cord injuries from brachial or lumbosacral plexus injuries, including cauda equina lesions, have recovered function from the reimplantation spinal cord surgery. This relatively less complicated injury, compared to a "classical" transverse spinal cord lesion, is obviously advantageous regarding chances for recovery.

The conus medullaris is the finely tapered distal or caudal end of the spinal cord. Cauda equina and conus medullaris forms of spinal cord injury relate to functions served by the sacral outflow, causing flaccid paralysis or paraplegia, autonomic dysfunction with an atonic bladder, and often severe intractable pain. A transverse lesion of the conus medullaris would mostly affect the lower motoneurons and CNS parts of the peripheral sensory neurons, together with nervous control over bladder and bowel function. A transverse caudal spinal cord injury at conus level has therefore many similarities with the root avulsion or the longitudinal type of spinal cord injury, and could in the future be considered for a similar type of surgical strategy. Avulsed roots would be implanted cranial to the site of the transverse spinal cord lesion in order to reverse lower extremity paralysis with return of locomotion, and reinnervate pelvic targets to reverse bladder and bowel dysfunction. Experimental surgery has been performed that has demonstrated functional return after such procedures (Liu *et al.* 1999; Tadie *et al.* 2002).

This book has described the first step in the direction to treat severe intraspinal nerve and spinal cord injuries. In order to reach further, to recover useful function and to alleviate pain, it is of course necessary to pursue research and development of basic and clinical science. Surgical and imaging refinements are also obligatory to achieve a full or near-normal functional restitution after brachial plexus and lumbosacral plexus avulsion injuries with minimal risks and efforts for the patient. A number of already available pharmaceutical substances, molecular products, and cellular therapies will be applied in the future to not only continue the achievement of recovery of injuries at the spinal cord surface, but also help find a cure for the more complete spinal cord injuries.

References

Al-Majed AA, Neumann CM, Brushart TM, Gordon T, Brief electrical stimulation promotes, the speed and accuracy of motor axonal regeneration, *J Neurosci* **20**:2602–2608, 2000.

Bergerot A, Shortland P, Anand P *et al.*, Co-treatment with riluzole and GDNF is necessary for functional recovery after ventral root avulsion injury, *Exp Neurol* **187**:359–366, 2004.

Berman JS, Anand P, Chin L *et al.*, Pain relief from preganglionic injury to the brachial plexus by late intercostal nerve transfer, *J Bone Joint Surg* **78**:759–760, 1996.

Berman JS, Birch R, Anand P, Pain following brachial plexus injury with spinal cord root avulsion and the effect of surgery, *Pain* **75**:199–207, 1998.

Blits B, Carlstedt T, Ruitenberg MJ *et al.*, Rescue and sprouting of motoneurons following ventral root avulsion and reimplantation combined with intraspinal adeno-associated viral vector-mediated expression of glial cell line–derived neurotrophic factor or brain-derived neurotrophic factor, *Exp Neurol* **189**:303–316, 2004.

Bradbury EJ, Moon LDF, Popat RJ *et al.*, Chondroitinase ABC promotes functional recovery after spinal cord injury, *Nature* **416**:637–640, 2002.

Brushart TME, Seiler WA, Selective reinnervation of distal motor stumps by peripheral motor axons, *Exp Neurol* **97**:289–300, 1987.

Carlstedt T, Regenerating axons from nerve terminals at astrocytes, *Brain Res* **347**:188–191, 1985.

Carlstedt T, Anand P, Hallin R *et al.*, Spinal nerve root repair and reimplantation of avulsed ventral roots into the spinal cord after brachial plexus injury, *J Neurosurg* **93**:237–247, 2000.

Carlstedt T, Anand P, Htut M *et al.*, Restoration of hand function and so called "breathing arm" after intraspinal repair of C5–T1 brachial plexus avulsion injury, *Neurosurg Focus* **16**:article 7, 2004.

Carlstedt T, Lindå H, Cullheim S, Risling M, Reinnervation of hind limb muscles after ventral root avulsion and implantation in the lumbar spinal cord of the adult rat, *Acta Physiol Scand* **128**:645–646, 1986.

Clowry GJ, Vrbova G, Observations on the development of transplanted embryonic ventral horn neurones grafted into adult rat spinal cord and connected to skeletal muscle implants via a peripheral nerve, *Exp Brain Res* **91**:249–258, 1992.

Cullheim S, Carlstedt T, Lindå H *et al.*, Motoneurons reinnervate skeletal muscle after ventral root implantation into the spinal cord of the cat, *Neuroscience* **29**:725–733, 1989.

Doble A, The pharmacology and mechanism of action of riluzole, *Neurology* **47**:233–241, 1996.

Fawcett J, Asher RA, The glial scar and central nervous system repair, *Brain Res Bull* **49**:377–391, 1999.

Giardino R, Fini M, Aldini NN *et al.*, Polyactive bioabsorbable polymers for guided tissue regeneration, *J Trauma Inj Infect Crit Care* **47**:303–308, 1999.

Guenot M, Bullies J, Rospars JP *et al.*, Single-unit analysis of the dorsal horn in patients with neuropathic pain, *J Clin Neurophysiol* **20**:143–150, 2003.

Hains BC, Klein JP, Saab CY *et al.*, Upregulation of sodium channel Nav 1.3 and functional involvement in neuronal hyperexcitability associated with central neuropathic pain after spinal cord injury, *J Neurosci* **23**:8881–8892, 2003.

Li L, Wu W, Lin LF *et al.*, Rescue of adult mouse motoneurons from injury-induced cell death by glial cell line–derived neurotrophic factor, *Proc Natl Acad Sci U S A* **92**:9771–9775, 1995.

Li Y, Carlstedt T, Berthold CH, Raisman G, Interaction of transplanted olfactory-ensheathing cells and host astrocytic processes provides a bridge for axons to regenerate across the dorsal root entry zone, *Exp Neurol* **188**:300–308, 2004.

Li Y, Decherchi P, Raisman G, Transplantation of olfactory ensheathing cells into spinal cord lesions restores breathing and climbing, *J Neurosci* **23**:727–731, 2003.

Li Y, Field PM, Raisman G, Repair of adult rat corticospinal tract by transplants of olfactory ensheathing cells, *Science* **277**:2000–2002, 1997.

Li Y, Raisman G, Schwann cells induce sprouting in motor and sensory axons in the adult rat spinal cord, *J Neurosci* **14**:4050–4063, 1994.

Liu S, Kadi K, Boisset N *et al.*, Reinnervation of denervated lumbar ventral roots and their target muscle by thoracic spinal motoneurons via an implanted nerve autograft in adult rats after spinal cord injury, *J Neurosci Res* **56**:506–517, 1999.

Madison RD, Archibald SJ, Lacin R, Krarup C, Factors contributing to preferential motor reinnervation in the primate nervous system, *J Neurosci* **19**:11007–11016, 1999.

Mattsson P, Aldskogius H, Svensson M, Nimodipine-induced improved survival rate of facial motor neurons following intracranial transection of the facial nerve in the adult rat, *J Neurosurg* **90**:760–765, 1999.

Morgenstern DA, Asher RA, Naidu M *et al.*, Expression and glycanation of the NG2 proteoglycan in developing, adult, and damaged peripheral nerve, *Mol Cell Neurosci* **24**:787–802, 2003.

Novikov L, Novikova L, Kellerth JO, Brain-derived neurotrophic factor promotes axonal regeneration and long-term survival of adult rat spinal motoneurons *in vivo*, *Neuroscience* **79**:765–774, 1997.

Ovelmen-Levitt J, Abnormal physiology of the dorsal horn as related to the deafferentation syndrome, *Appl Neurophysiol* **51**:104–116, 1988.

Priestley JV, Ramer MS, King VR *et al.*, Stimulating regeneration in the damaged spinal cord, *J Physiol Paris* **96**:123–133, 2002.

Raisman G, A promising therapeutic approach to spinal cord repair, *J R Soc Med* **96**:259–261, 2003.

Ramer MS, Duraisingam I, Priestley JV, McMahon SB, Two-tiered inhibition at the dorsal root entry zone, *J Neurosci* **21**:2651–2660, 2001.

Ramer MS, Priestley JV, McMahon SB, Functional regeneration of sensory axons into the adult spinal cord, *Nature* **403**:312–316, 2000.

Roth G, Reinnervation dans la paralysie plexulaire brachiale obstétricale, *J Neurol Sci* **58**:103–115, 1983.

Tadie M, Liu S, Robert R, Partial return of motor function in paralyzed legs after surgical bypass of the lesion site by nerve autografts three years after spinal cord injury, *J Neurotrauma* **19**:909–916, 2002.

Watkins L, Maier S, Glia: a novel drug discovery target for clinical pain, *Nat Rev Drug Discov* **2**:973–985, 2003.

Index